MEDITERRANEAN 300 RECIPES COOBOOK

Table of Contents

Drinks

Cranberry Drink

INGREDIENTS

- Fresh cranberries 500 g
- Beets 1 piece
- Apple 2.5 kg
- Celery 1 stalk
- Lemon ½ pieces

COOKING INSTRUCTION 25 MINUTES

1. Squeeze the juice from all the **INGREDIENTS**.
2. Mix well and serve in a large jug.

Apple drink with lemon

INGREDIENTS

- Green apples 2 pieces
- Lemon 1 piece
- Sugar 2 tablespoons
- Water 5 cups
- Honeyto taste
- Raisinsto taste

COOKING INSTRUCTION 15 MINUTES

1. Peel the apples and remove the core.
2. Prepare a decoction of the peel and core, boiling for 10 minutes.
3. Strain the broth, add chopped apples, thin slices of lemon, sugar.
4. You can add honey or raisins to taste.

Ginger drink with cucumbers and mint

INGREDIENTS

- Mineral water 5 l
- Fresh mint 1 bunch
- Lime 1 piece
- Lemon 2 pieces
- Fresh ginger 50 g
- Honey 2 tablespoons
- Cucumbers 2 pieces

COOKING INSTRUCTION 20 MINUTES + 5 MINUTES

1. Add 3-4 cm of grated fresh ginger root to a large pot of mineral or any other quality water (you can also taste more), a large bunch of fresh mint, thinly sliced lime, squeeze the juice of a whole lemon (squeezed halves there) and thinly sliced cucumbers, add 2 tablespoons of honey (I love it to be savory).
2. Infuse the drink at room temperature for several hours, then send it overnight in the refrigerator. In the afternoon, strain, add a few fresh circles of cucumber, lime, lemon and mint.

Apple and nut drink

INGREDIENTS

- Milk 1 cup
- Orange juice 1 cup
- Vanilla Yogurt 1 cup
- Peanut butter 2 teaspoons
- Crushed ice 2 cups

COOKING INSTRUCTION 15 MINUTES
1. Mix half of each ingredient in a blender, stir the mixture until it becomes homogeneous. Repeat with the remaining **INGREDIENTS**. Pour the drink into glasses and serve.

Orange Peel Drink

INGREDIENTS
- Oranges 3 pieces
- Citric acid 3 teaspoons
- Sugar 1.5 cups
- Water 3.5 L

COOKING INSTRUCTION 30 MINUTES + 1 DAY
1. Soak for a day the peel of oranges along with the white part, placing them in a 0.5 liter jar of cold boiled water and citric acid.
2. Put the jar in the refrigerator.
3. Then bring to a boil the sugar with the remaining amount of water.
4. Cool the syrup, grind the crusts from the can through a meat grinder. Store liquid in the jar.
5. When the water with sugar has cooled, add crushed crusts there and filter by pouring them into bottles or jars and refrigerate.

Banana and Tahini Drink

INGREDIENTS
- Bananas 1 piece
- Tahini 2 tablespoons

COOKING INSTRUCTION 5 MINUTES
1. In a blender, beat the chopped banana, tahini and 1 cup of water. Serve.
2. If the mixture is very thick, add a little water, and if it is very thin, add a little banana.

Barley Lemon Drink

INGREDIENTS
- Lemon 2 pieces
- Cane sugar 50 g
- Pearl barley 125 g

COOKING INSTRUCTION 30 MINUTES
1. Grate zest with lemons and transfer to a bowl. Add sugar.
2. Rinse the pearl barley and transfer to the zest, pour 1.2 liters of hot water (boiling water). Mix well and let cool.
3. In the cooled mass, squeeze the juice from the lemons, strain through a sieve and cool. Pour into tall glasses with ice.

Mexican Refreshment

INGREDIENTS
- Vanilla Rice Milk 1 cup
- Vanilla ice cream 1 cup
- Ground cinnamon ½ teaspoon

COOKING INSTRUCTION 30 MINUTES
1. In a blender, mix rice milk, ice cream, and 0.25 teaspoons of cinnamon. Beat and serve immediately, sprinkling with the remaining

Apple Juice Coffee Drink

INGREDIENTS
- Water 100 ml
- Apple juice 50 g
- Natural coffee 15 g
- Milk 20 ml

COOKING INSTRUCTION 5 MINUTES

1. Mix apple juice with milk and add the resulting mass to the prepared strained coffee.

Drink from the leaves and berries of lingonberry

INGREDIENTS

- Lingonberry 100 g
- Lingonberry leaves 20 g
- Water 1 L
- Honey 3 tablespoons

COOKING INSTRUCTION 10 MINUTES

1. Boil water, brew lingonberry leaves.
2. Rub the lingonberry berries through a strainer.
3. Add honey to the kettle, or individually to each cup.

Broccoli, Celery and Cabbage Drink

INGREDIENTS

- Broccoli cabbage 2 pieces
- Celery stalk ½ pieces
- ½ bunchfeed cabbage
- Young carrots 2 pieces
- Apple ¼ pieces
- Ice ½ cup

COOKING INSTRUCTION 10 MINUTES

1. Put all the **INGREDIENTS** in a blender or combine and grind.
2. Add 0.25 cups of water and beat, alternating high and low speeds.
3. Serve immediately

Rice drink from Chile (Horchata)

ENERGY VALUE PER PORTION
CALORIE CONTENT166KCAL
SQUIRRELS 5.3 GRAM
FATS 13.6 GRAM
CARBOHYDRATES 6.1 GRAM
INGREDIENTS

- Poppy 75 g
- Cinnamon sticks 1 piece
- Honey 2 tablespoons
- Vanilla Pod ¼ g
- Water 4 cups
- Lime zest 1 tablespoon
- Almonds 65 g

COOKING INSTRUCTION 25 MINUTES

1. Rub the zest of 2 limes, put it in a container (for example, a jug).
2. In a blender, mix almonds, water, honey and poppy seeds.
3. Filter the resulting fluid through cheesecloth and pour into a jug.
4. Add the cinnamon stick and cover.
5. Put the vessel in the refrigerator for infusion. It is better to insist all night, but it can be 4-6 hours.
6. Before serving, filter again.

Lemon drink with ginger ale and mint

ENERGY VALUE PER PORTION
CALORIE CONTENT 354 KCAL
SQUIRRELS 2.1 GRAM
FATS 0.2 GRAM

CARBOHYDRATES 87.7 GRAM
INGREDIENTS
- SERVINGS
- Lemon juice 2 cups
- Sugar ¾ cup
- Water 4 cups
- Ginger Ale 2 L
- 15 mint leaves
- Lemon Sorbetto taste
- Lemon 2 pieces

COOKING INSTRUCTION 40 MINUTES

1. Mix lemon juice and sugar and mix until sugar dissolves. Add water and refrigerate for 30 minutes.
2. In a large punch bowl, mix the lemon mixture and ginger ale. Add the balls of sorbet, sliced into thin slices of lemons and mint. Serve right away.

Invigorating Spinach

ENERGY VALUE PER PORTION
CALORIE CONTENT 112 KCAL
SQUIRRELS 7.1 GRAM
FATS 1 GRAM
CARBOHYDRATES 19.8 GRAM
INGREDIENTS
- Spinach 280 g
- Tomatoes 4 pieces
- 2 carrots
- Lemon ¼ pieces
- Cucumbers 1 piece

COOKING INSTRUCTION 15 MINUTES

1. Squeeze the juice from all the **INGREDIENTS** and serve immediately.

Herbal Tropic Warming Drink

INGREDIENTS
- Kaffir lime 3 g
- Rosemary 1 sprig
- Pineapple puree 100 g
- Vanilla Syrup 80 ml
- Pineapple juice 210 ml

COOKING INSTRUCTION 10 MINUTES

1. Mix kafir lime, a sprig of rosemary, pineapple puree and pineapple juice, cream soda syrup.
2. Heat the resulting drink and add boiling water.
3. Bon appetit!

Drink with anon fruits

ENERGY VALUE PER PORTION
CALORIE CONTENT 226 KCAL
SQUIRRELS 3.6 GRAM
FATS 1,1 GRAM
CARBOHYDRATES 57.4 GRAM
INGREDIENTS
- Pears 5 pieces
- Blackberry 190 g
- Frozen anon fruits 1 cup

COOKING INSTRUCTION 20 MINUTES

1. Gently squeeze juice from pears and berries.
2. In a blender, mix juice with frozen anon fruits and serve.

Wheat Sprout Drink (Reggelac)

ENERGY VALUE PER PORTION
CALORIE CONTENT 17 KCAL
SQUIRRELS 0.7 GRAM
FATS 0.1 GRAM
CARBOHYDRATES 3.6 GRAM
INGREDIENTS

- Water 6 glasses
- Wheat Sprouts ½ cup

COOKING INSTRUCTION 1 HOUR + 5 MINUTES

1. Grind the seedlings. Place in a 2-3 liter jar or bottle, pour water and cover with gauze to breathe. Leave on for 3 days. After 4 days, the drink is ready (in hot weather earlier). Strain it into another container ... and drink it!

Tema special drink

ENERGY VALUE PER PORTION
CALORIE CONTENT 257 KCAL
SQUIRRELS 0.1 GRAM
FATS 0 GRAM
CARBOHYDRATES 32.6 GRAM
INGREDIENTS

- Golden rum 30 ml
- Watermelon pulpto taste
- Limoncello 30 ml
- Honey syrup 30 ml
- Lime juice 30 ml

COOKING INSTRUCTION 5 MINUTES

1. Cut the watermelon into thin slices (slices).
2. Watermelon slices are vertically laid out in a large glass "bowl", then whipped in a shaker: golden rum, limoncello, honey syrup and lime juice and poured on top onto watermelon slices so that they are saturated with this cocktail.

Kefir drink with cucumber, dill and garlic

ENERGY VALUE PER PORTION
CALORIE CONTENT 89 KCAL
SQUIRRELS 5.7 GRAM
FATS 3,1 GRAM
CARBOHYDRATES 9.5 GRAM
INGREDIENTS

- Kefir 300 ml
- Dillto taste
- Garlic 1 clove
- Sea saltto taste
- Cucumbers 1 piece

COOKING INSTRUCTION 15 MINUTES

1. Wash and chop vegetables and herbs arbitrarily (instead of or along with dill, you can take parsley and / or celery), put everything in a glass for a blender, add half the chilled kefir (or sour milk), but then you need to dilute it with mineral water so that it is not thick, or vice versa, add 1-3 tablespoons of cottage cheese to turn into a cottage cheese salad, but then it will be another dish), and beat everything until smooth.

2. Add salt and beat everything again, until the **INGREDIENTS** are completely small.

3. Pour into cups (the edges of which can be decorated with grains of salt).

4. Serve cold.

Chocolate Nut Coffee Drink

ENERGY VALUE PER PORTION
CALORIE CONTENT 600 KCAL
SQUIRRELS 13.9 GRAM
FATS 56.9 GRAM
CARBOHYDRATES 8.7 GRAM
INGREDIENTS

- Milk chocolateto taste
- Water 2 cups
- Hazelnuts 85 g
- Freshly brewed coffee ½ cup
- Cocoa Powderto taste
- Vanilla sugarto taste
- Sugarto taste
- Ground cinnamonto taste

COOKING INSTRUCTION 15 MINUTES

1. We make nut milk. Pour nuts into a blender and fill with water. It is better to soak them at night if, for example, you want to drink this drink in the morning. I had only hazelnuts, you can use almonds instead. We prepare milk for about 5-7 minutes, then filter it through a fine sieve or gauze.

2. We make coffee. Coffee needs good, rich, otherwise the taste of nuts will completely kill him. I brewed a Nespresso 6 coffee maker.

3. Add grated chocolate to our milk, stir, I am a big lover of chocolate, so I added a lot. Put in the microwave for 1.5–2 minutes.

4. In a clean blender, pour cinnamon, vanilla sugar and ordinary (if you want), cocoa (if you want more chocolate flavor - add more).

5. Pour milk and coffee into a blender, beat well and you're done!

Champagne carbonated drink

ENERGY VALUE PER PORTION
CALORIE CONTENT 662 KCAL
SQUIRRELS 3,5 GRAM
FATS 2 GRAM
CARBOHYDRATES 98.3 GRAM
INGREDIENTS

- Water 3 cups
- Cranberry juice 2.7 kg
- Lemonade Concentrate 330 ml
- Dry champagne 1.5 l

COOKING INSTRUCTION 30 MINUTES

1. In the decanter, mix cold water, cranberry juice and concentrated lemonade. Mix well and pour in chilled champagne. Gently mix and serve.

Apple Nutts Warm Drink

ENERGY VALUE PER PORTION
CALORIE CONTENT 193 KCAL
SQUIRRELS 3 GRAM
FATS 2,8 GRAM
CARBOHYDRATES 40.3 GRAM
INGREDIENTS

- Caramel Syrup 75 ml

- Freshly squeezed apple juice 150 ml
- Hazelnut milk 300 ml
- Orange syrup 75 ml

COOKING INSTRUCTION 30 MINUTES

1. Mix caramel-orange syrup with freshly squeezed apple juice and hazelnut milk
2. Heat the resulting drink before serving
3. Bon appetit!

Winter warming drink

ENERGY VALUE PER PORTION
CALORIE CONTENT 34 KCAL
SQUIRRELS 0.3 GRAM
FATS 0.7 GRAM
CARBOHYDRATES 6.3 GRAM
INGREDIENTS

- Ginger Syrup 100 ml
- Sea buckthorn 4 teaspoons
- Pineapple Juice 150 ml

COOKING INSTRUCTION 10 MINUTES

1. Grind sea buckthorn, add pineapple juice and ginger syrup.
2. Mix the resulting consistency and serve with the addition of boiling water (200 ml)
3. Bon appetit!.

Ginger drink

INGREDIENTS

- Lemon 1 piece
- Fresh ginger 1 piece
- Honey 1 tablespoon
- Anise (star anise)to taste
- Boiling water 1 cup

COOKING INSTRUCTION 10 MINUTES

1. Cut 10 thin slices from fresh ginger root. Put in a large glass, add 1 slice of fresh lemon. You can also add anise or cinnamon to taste. Pour boiling water and cover, wait about 10-15 minutes.
2. After that, add honey to taste (immediately it is better not to add honey, because it loses all the beneficial properties at temperatures above 60 degrees). You can use a mug with a lid or a thermos.

Berry drink

INGREDIENTS

- Fresh cranberries 150 g
- Sugar 120 g
- Water 1 L

COOKING INSTRUCTION 1 HOUR

1. Squeeze the squeezes with hot water, boil at low boil for 5-8 minutes and let it brew for 25-30 minutes.
2. Strain the broth, squeeze, add sugar to the broth and stir it until it is completely dissolved.
3. Then pour in the juice, strain and cool again.
4. Rinse fresh berries and squeeze juice.

Cocoa Energy Drink

INGREDIENTS

- Water 30 ml
- Cocoa 2 teaspoons
- Instant coffee 1 teaspoon
- Sugar 2 teaspoons

- Chicken egg 1 piece
- Milk 400 ml
- Wheat sprouts 1 teaspoon

COOKING INSTRUCTION 10 MINUTES

1. Pour cocoa and coffee with boiling water, stir.
2. Add sugar, egg, wheat and milk.
3. Pour everything into a blender and beat at high speed.

Sea buckthorn and ginger drink

INGREDIENTS

- Sea buckthorn 1 cup
- Ginger 50 g
- Honey 2 tablespoons
- Water 1 L

COOKING INSTRUCTION 10 MINUTES

1. Ginger cut into thin slices. If you like the more spicy taste of the drink, it is better to ginger on a coarse grater.
2. Boil water.
3. Wipe the sea buckthorn through a fine strainer into the kettle. Throw chopped ginger into the water.
4. In the slightly cooled drink, add honey to taste ..

Coconut drink

INGREDIENTS

- Coconut ½ pieces
- Bananas 1 piece
- Lime ½ pieces
- Vanilla Pod 1 piece
- Oranges 2 pieces

COOKING INSTRUCTION 20 MINUTES

1. Put milk and coconut pulp, banana, lime juice, orange juice and a slice of vanilla in a blender.
2. Grind until smooth.

Coconut and Avocado Drink

INGREDIENTS

- Coconut 1 piece
- Avocado 1 piece
- Greens 1 bunch

COOKING INSTRUCTION 15 MINUTES

1. Pour coconut milk into a blender.
2. Halve the coconut and take out the pulp. Add to blender.
3. Add avocado and greens and beat until smooth

Italian Coffee and Chocolate Drink (Affogato)

INGREDIENTS

- Espresso 240 ml
- cupcoffee liquor
- Chocolate ice cream 8 tablespoons

COOKING INSTRUCTION 30 MINUTES

1. In the decanter, mix coffee and liquor. Place the ice cream in 8 small cups and pour the coffee. Serve right away.

Cranberry drink

INGREDIENTS

- Anise (star anise) 1 piece
- Frozen Cranberries 250 g
- Water 2 L
- Sugar 5 tablespoons
- Cinnamon sticks 1 piece
- Cloves 3 pieces

COOKING INSTRUCTION 3 HOURS + 5 MINUTES

1. Boil water with sugar and spices.
2. Grind cranberries.
3. Put the resulting berry puree in boiling syrup, stir and remove from the stove. Leave for a couple of hours until completely cooled.
4. Strain, pour into a jug.

Coconut Drink

INGREDIENTS

- Apple 1 piece
- Dates 95 g
- Raisins 95 g
- Almonds 80 g
- Coconut Pulp 100 g
- Ground cinnamon 2 teaspoons
- Ginger juice 1 teaspoon
- Nutmegpinch
- Ground clovepinch
- Coconut milk 2 cups

COOKING INSTRUCTION 15 MINUTES

1. Soak nuts and dates for 8-12 hours in water.
2. Put all the **INGREDIENTS** in a blender and chop until smooth.

Orange drink

INGREDIENTS

- Sugar 250 g
- Oranges 1 piece
- Citric acid 7 g
- Water 2.2 L

COOKING INSTRUCTION 30 MINUTES + 8 HOURS

1. Wash the orange, scald it with boiling water to remove the bitterness, wipe it dry and put it in the freezer for 3-4 hours, or better, overnight. Can be pre-cut into 4 parts.
2. Remove the orange from the freezer and scroll through the meat grinder or in the combine.
3. Pour the resulting mass into 750 ml of boiled water and let it brew for 10 minutes.
4. Strain everything through a colander, then through 4 layers of gauze.
5. Add 250 grams of sugar, 7 grams of citric acid and the remaining 1500 ml of water to the strained juice.
6. Pour into a glass container, insist an hour and you can try.

Blueberry and Parsley Drink

INGREDIENTS

- Parsley ½ bunch
- Blueberries ½ cup
- Ginger Root 1 piece

- Lemon ¼ pieces
- Mineral water ½ cup

COOKING INSTRUCTION 10 MINUTES

1. Grind all the **INGREDIENTS** in a blender to a cream. Drink for breakfast.

Apple cucumber drink

INGREDIENTS
- Lemon zest 1 teaspoon
- Cucumbers 1 piece
- Apple 3 pieces

COOKING INSTRUCTION 15 MINUTES

1. Squeeze the juice from all the **INGREDIENTS**, mix well and serve immediately.

Persimmon drink

INGREDIENTS
- Almonds 320 g
- Dates 6 pieces
- Mineral water 3 cups
- Persimmon 3 pieces
- Nutmeg ½ teaspoon
- Ground cinnamon ½ teaspoon
- Cardamom ¼ teaspoon

COOKING INSTRUCTION 15 MINUTES + 12 HOURS

1. Soak the nuts for 8-12 hours in water.
2. In a blender, mix nuts, dates and water until creamy.
3. Put the mixture in cheesecloth and let drain in a bowl.
4. Return the almond milk to the blender and add the rest of the **INGREDIENTS**.
5. Stir well for about 30 seconds and serve.

Blue Hawaii Drink

INGREDIENTS
- Bacardi rum 30 ml
- Liqueur "Blue Curacao" 30 ml
- Pineapple juice 60 ml
- Sugar Syrup 30 ml
- Lemon juice 30 ml
- Pineapple 1 piece
- Mint leaves 1 piece
- Cocktail Cherry 1 piece

COOKING INSTRUCTION 5 MINUTES

1. Mix with ice all the **INGREDIENTS** in a portioned bowl.
2. Garnish with a pineapple segment, a leaf of mint, a cocktail cherry and straws

Nutritious strawberry drink

INGREDIENTS
- Almonds 80 g
- Strawberry 80 g
- Bananas 1 piece
- Blue-green algae 1 teaspoon
- Water 1 cup
- Spicesto taste
- Vanilla 1 teaspoon

- Sea saltto taste

COOKING INSTRUCTION 10 MINUTES + 12 HOURS

1. Soak the almonds overnight in water.
2. In a blender, beat all the **INGREDIENTS** until creamy. Drink in small sips.

Dandelion drink

INGREDIENTS

Dandelion Leaves 20 Pieces
Apple 2 pieces
5 celery stalk

COOKING INSTRUCTION 15 MINUTES

1. Squeeze the juice from all the **INGREDIENTS** and mix well.

White-blue-red drink

INGREDIENTS

- Crushed iceto taste
- Cranberry juice 1 cup
- Gatorade blue drink 1 glass
- Diet sprite 1 cup

COOKING INSTRUCTION 30 MINUTES PRINT

1. Fill tall glasses with ice.
2. Fill the glasses a third with cranberry juice, then gently pour the blue drink and then fill the third part with the sprite.

Coconut Nut Drink

INGREDIENTS

- Coconut 3 pieces
- Cashew ½ cup
- Macadamia nuts ½ cup
- Dates 7 pieces
- Ginger Root 1 piece
- Ground cinnamon ½ teaspoon
- Cardamom ¼ teaspoon
- Ground black pepper ¼ teaspoon
- Ground clovepinch

COOKING INSTRUCTION 15 MINUTES + 12 HOURS

1. Soak the nuts for 8-12 hours in water.
2. In a blender, mix the flesh of 2 coconuts, 3 cups of coconut milk, nuts and other **INGREDIENTS** until creamy.
3. For a thinner consistency, dilute with water or coconut milk.

Orange and berry drink with ginger

INGREDIENTS

- Ginger Root 1 piece
- Oranges 4 pieces
- Fresh berries 110 g

COOKING INSTRUCTION 15 MINUTES

1. Squeeze the juice from all the **INGREDIENTS** and mix well. Serve immediately.

Berry drink

INGREDIENTS
- Dates 5 pieces
- Bananas 2 pieces
- Strawberry 150 g
- Raspberry 90 g
- Orange juice 1 cup

COOKING INSTRUCTION 15 MINUTES
1. Soak dates for 20 minutes in water.
2. In a blender, mix 1 banana, dates and the water in which they were soaked, berries and orange juice.

Frappuccino Cold Coffee Drink (Frappuccino)

INGREDIENTS
- Black coffee 150 ml
- Milk 150 ml
- Sugar 1.5 tablespoons
- Chocolate syrup 3 tablespoons
- Ice 350 g
- Whipped creamto taste

COOKING INSTRUCTION 10 MINUTES
1. Pour cold coffee into a blender.
2. Then add milk, 1.5 tablespoons of sugar, 3 tablespoons of syrup, 350-400 ml of ice.
3. Beat the **INGREDIENTS** in a blender for 1 minute.
4. Pour into a large glass, a glass (wherever you want).
5. Pour whipped cream on top.
6. Pour over the cream with chocolate syrup to taste.

Refreshing watermelon drink

INGREDIENTS
- Sugar 1 tablespoon
- Lime juice 2 tablespoons
- Watermelon Pulp 3 cups
- Crushed ice 1 cup
- Water ½ cup

COOKING INSTRUCTION 30 MINUTES
1. In a blender, mix the pulp of watermelon, lime juice, sugar, crushed ice and water. Beat until smooth and serve immediately.

Papaya, Almond and Cardamom Drink

INGREDIENTS
- Cardamom boxes 4 pieces
- Papaya 1 piece
- Almonds 160 g
- Water 1 cup

COOKING INSTRUCTION 10 MINUTES + 6 HOURS
1. Soak the almonds for 6 hours in water.
2. In a blender, chop the almonds with 1 cup of water. Strain.
3. Remove the seeds from the cardamom boxes and place in a blender.
4. Add chopped papaya and almond milk.
5. Grind until smooth. Add water as needed.

SAUCES AND MARINADES

Pickled garlic

INGREDIENTS
- Garlic 250 g
- Salt 1 tablespoon
- Sherry vinegar 50 ml
- Sugar 50 g
- White Wine Vinegar 50 ml

COOKING INSTRUCTION 20 MINUTES

1. Peel the garlic cloves, put in a saucepan with boiling salted water and, stirring, cook for three to four minutes to remove the bitterness. Drain and transfer the garlic into a half-liter jar.

2. In a saucepan, heat a mixture of two vinegar, sherry and white wine, water and sugar (vinegar should be as much as sugar and water together), stir and wait for the sugar to dissolve. Pour the garlic with the hot mixture of vinegar, clog the jar and let stand for at least a week.

Banya cauda

INGREDIENTS
- Extra virgin olive oil 200 ml
- Anchovies 15 pieces
- Garlic 6 cloves
- Butter 130 g
- Ground black pepperto taste
- Saltto taste

COOKING INSTRUCTION 30 MINUTES

1. Very finely chopped garlic and anchovies.

2. In a skillet over low heat, heat olive oil with anchovies.

3. After a couple of minutes add the garlic. Stir constantly.

4. In another minute, add butter to the resulting unclear mass. When it breaks a little bit, drive it into the whisk.

5. Taste, pepper and salt to taste. Serve in a heated bowl with bread and any fresh vegetables.

Pickled radish

INGREDIENTS

Radish 1 kg
Red wine vinegar 50 ml
Sugar 50 g
White Wine Vinegar 50 ml
Water 100 ml

COOKING INSTRUCTION 50 MINUTES

1. Wash the radish, cut the tops (small green cuttings from the tops can be left), cut in half and lay tightly in a liter jar.

2. In a saucepan, heat a mixture of two vinegars, red and white wine, water and sugar (as in previous recipes, the ratio of the mixture of two types of vinegar should be one to one with water and sugar). Wait for the sugar to completely dissolve, then let the resulting mixture cool (you must not pour hot so that the radish does not cook) and fill it with a jar to the top. Cork it and stand for three days.

Aivar

INGREDIENTS
- Red bell pepper 1 kg
- Eggplant 300 g
- Garlic 5 cloves
- Vegetable oil 20 ml

- Olive oil 60 ml
- White wine vinegar 1 tablespoon
- Saltto taste
- Ground black pepperto taste
- Sugarto taste

COOKING INSTRUCTION 2 HOURS PRINT

1. Pierce the eggplant with a fork in several places, wrap it with foil and send it to the oven, preheated to 180 degrees, together with peppers greased with vegetable oil for 30–40 minutes. The eggplant should become soft, and the skin of peppers blacken.

2. Put the peppers in a large bowl and cover with a lid or cling film. Remove the eggplant from the foil. Allow the vegetables to cool for 10-15 minutes.

3. Cut the eggplant along one side, open and scoop up the pulp with a spoon. Peppers peel and seeds, chop coarsely. Punch vegetables in a blender with garlic, vinegar, oil, a teaspoon of salt and pepper until smooth.

4. Transfer the vegetable mass to a saucepan, bring to a boil and cook on low heat for 30 minutes. Season with salt, pepper and sugar to taste, remove from heat and let cool. Eat immediately or shift to a jar and store in the refrigerator for up to two weeks.

Curry sauce

INGREDIENTS
- 5 tablespoonssunflower oil
- Mustard Seeds 2 teaspoons
- Ginger 30 g
- Curry leaves 1 bunch
- Fenugreek 1 teaspoon
- Onion 3 heads
- Paprikato taste
- Turmeric 1 teaspoon
- Tomatoes 6 pieces
- Water 1 cup
- Salt 1 teaspoon
- Chili pepper 3 pieces
- Coconut milk 1 can

COOKING INSTRUCTION 20 MINUTES PRINT

1. Put a small stewpan on medium heat, add sunflower oil, mustard seeds, fenugreek and a handful of curry leaves. Mix gently.

2. Peel the chili seeds, cut into thin strips, put in a pan. Peel fresh ginger and grate. Add to pan and mix with other spices.

3. Chop the onion, add to the mixture, mix. Then add paprika and turmeric. Peel, chop and chop the tomatoes - for speed, this can be done in a blender. And also send to the pan.

4. Pour a glass of water into the pan, add salt, then coconut milk, mix gently. Leave the sauce for five minutes to boil over medium heat.

5. Pour cooked rice, fish or chicken with hot curry sauce and serve immediately. Or cool, refrigerate and store for a couple of days. And before serving, reheat well again.

Pickled carrots

INGREDIENTS
- Carrot 1 kg
- Sugar 50 g
- White Wine Vinegar 100 ml
- Chili pepper ½ pieces

COOKING INSTRUCTION 15 MINUTES

1. Wash the carrots, peel and cut into circles about 3 cm thick (you can also use quarters or otherwise, as long as the pieces are large).
2. Cut the half of the chili pepper into very thin rings. Pour water and vinegar in a 1: 2 ratio into a stewpan, add sugar and put on fire.
3. Add chili peppers and stir until sugar is completely dissolved in water and vinegar, or just let the liquid boil a little. After that, add chopped carrots to the stewpan and boil for another two minutes.
4. Then transfer the carrots to the jar and fill it to the top with liquid from the stewpan.

Satsebeli sauce

INGREDIENTS

- Walnuts 300 g
- Garlic ½ head
- Ground red pepper 1.5 teaspoons
- Cilantro 35 g
- Imereti saffron 1 teaspoon
- Pomegranate juice ¾ cup
- Saltto taste

COOKING INSTRUCTION 5 MINUTES

1. Crush nuts with pepper, salt, garlic and cilantro, add Imereti saffron.
2. The resulting mixture is gradually diluted with broth, rubbing all the time.
3. Then pour in the juice of unripe grapes, pomegranate or blackberry.

Caesar Salad Sauce

INGREDIENTS

- Egg yolk 1 piece
- Garlic 2 cloves
- Anchovies 4 pieces
- Salt 1 teaspoon
- Ground black pepper 1 teaspoon
- Worcestershire sauce 1 teaspoon
- Olive oil 150 ml
- Dijon mustard 1 teaspoon
- Lemon juice 1 tablespoon
- Grated Parmesan Cheese 50 g

COOKING INSTRUCTION 5 MINUTES

1. Beat the whisk with a whisk with egg yolk and salt in a deep bowl. While adding olive oil, beat the contents of the bowl into mayonnaise. After all the olive oil has been whipped, add lemon juice, ground pepper, Worcestershire sauce, crushed anchovy fillets, crushed garlic and grated parmesan to the sauce. Beat with a whisk and serve with any salad leaves, chicken meat and everything else edible.

Ranchero

INGREDIENTS

- Tomatoes 1 piece
- Cayenne pepperpinch
- Red bell pepper 1 piece
- Cocoa with chili ⅓ teaspoon
- Ground paprika 1 teaspoon
- Oreganopinch
- Concentrated tomato paste 1 teaspoon
- Cilantro 15 g
- Sugar 1 teaspoon
- Red onion 1 head

- Freshly ground black pepper to taste
- Garlic 3 cloves
- 1 tablespoon olive oil
- Cocoa pinch

COOKING INSTRUCTION 40 MINUTES

1. Remove the pulp from one large tomato, chop it coarsely. What remains on the skin - three millimeters - also cut into cubes. Chop onion finely. Peel and chop red pepper into small cubes. Remove the core from the cloves of garlic and chop. Divide all vegetables into two parts - two-thirds of each will be fried, the remaining third will need to be added at the end.

2. Put large pieces of chopped vegetables in a pan. Add cayenne pepper, dried paprika, oregano, cocoa chili, sugar, salt and pepper to taste. Passer, stirring constantly, over a hot fire until all this turns into a mess.

3. Stir in a teaspoon of vegetables with a slide of tomato paste.

4. Go through the vegetables with a hand blender, and then rub the resulting mashed potatoes through a sieve.

5. Stir in the sauce the remaining fresh vegetables, finely chopped cilantro and a pinch of dried cocoa.

Tomato Salsa

INGREDIENTS
- Tomatoes 4 pieces
- Tomato paste 2 tablespoons
- Red onion 1 head
- Carrot 100 g
- Celery 1 stalk
- Garlic 4 cloves
- Chili Sauce 4 Tbsp
- Tomato juice 100 ml
- Basil 20 g
- Olive oil 50 ml
- Red bell pepper 1 piece
- Butter 50 g
- Salt to taste

COOKING INSTRUCTION 1 HOUR 10 MINUTES

1. Finely chop the onion, garlic, celery and carrots and fry until soft in olive oil. Add finely chopped tomatoes (having previously removed the entrails from them), chopped bell peppers, tomato paste and tomato juice and simmer for five minutes.

2. Then add the sweet and spicy chili sauce and chopped basil, mix and simmer for another five minutes.

3. Pour the sauce into a blender, beat, then strain through a fine sieve and put on the fire again. Salt, cook until thickened. Remove from the heat and drive into the sauce with whisk ice butter, cut into small cubes.

Creamy a la Bearnez with cilantro

INGREDIENTS
- Butter 250 g
- Shallots 1 head
- White wine vinegar 2 tablespoons
- Egg yolk 3 pieces
- Cilantro 5 g
- Green Basil 5 g
- Salt to taste
- Ground black pepper to taste

COOKING INSTRUCTION 40 MINUTES

1. Put oil in a saucepan and put on fire. When it melts, remove the foam and carefully pour the upper transparent layer into another dish. The lower, creamy, is no longer useful.

2. Finely chop the shallots, temporarily set aside half, put the other in a saucepan, pour vinegar and put on fire. Evaporate, stirring until moisture is completely gone.

3. Beat three egg yolks and two tablespoons of water with a whisk in an emulsion. Stir in half the steamed onions. In a steam bath - you can just hold a bowl over a pot of boiling water - beat the sauce for about five minutes, until by consistency it looks like shaving foam. It is important not to overheat - so as not to get an omelet, so you can occasionally remove the bowl from the steam.

4. Gradually pour oil into the sauce, thoroughly whipping it after each new serving.

5. Finely chop the cilantro and green basil. Pour them into the sauce along with the remains of fresh shallots. Stir, salt and pepper to taste.

Berblan

INGREDIENTS

- Shallots 1 piece
- Butter 35 g
- White wine vinegar 2 tablespoons
- Cream 48% 200 ml
- Fish broth 1 tablespoon
- Tomatoes ¼ pieces

COOKING INSTRUCTION 20 MINUTES

1. Finely chop the onion and fry in butter until transparent. Pour vinegar and simmer, simmer until all liquid has evaporated. Then add the broth - and evaporate it.

2. Add fat cream to the stewpan. Stew until the cream thickens, and then pour 30 grams of oil into them.

3. Cut the lean meat from the tomato, cut it into small cubes and mix in the sauce.

Bordelez

INGREDIENTS

Dry red wine 300 ml
Thyme 1 bunch
Shallots 2 heads
Beef broth 500 ml
Black pepper peas 10 pieces
Butter 50 g

COOKING INSTRUCTION 25 MINUTES

1. Pour wine into a deep stewpan and put a large bunch of thyme and roughly chopped onions. Put on fire and leave to boil for five to seven minutes over high heat.

2. At the same time, in another stewpan, also keep on a light fire for five to seven minutes half a liter of beef broth. Then pour the broth into the wine and evaporate the mixture for another fifteen minutes, so that the onion has time to boil, and the consistency is reached close to the syrup.

3. Strain the sauce through a fine sieve into another saucepan. Put it on fire. Divide the oil into five to six pieces and add one to the wine, after each serving, slightly rotate the saucepan over a fire until the oil dissolves.

Sofrito

INGREDIENTS

- Onion 1 kg
- Tomatoes 6 pieces
- Olive oil 250 ml
- Garlic 2 cloves

COOKING INSTRUCTION 2 HOURS 45 MINUTES

1. First chop the onion into very thin half rings, and then into small cubes. Grate the tomatoes (plum-shaped or simply not very large - about a hundred grams each) until they are mashed, having previously removed all the flesh from them with a spoon or knife.

2. Heat the olive oil in a pan and simmer the onions in it for one and a half to two hours at the lowest heat. After that add tomatoes to the onion and simmer another twenty to thirty minutes; then add the finely chopped cloves of garlic and then simmer another five minutes.

3. Remove from heat, transfer to a jar and clog it.

INGREDIENTS

- Tomatoes 4 pieces
- Basil 2 stalks
- Mozzarella Cheese 125 g
- Olives 8 pieces
- Extra virgin olive oil 2 tablespoons
- Crutons 30 g
- Cream 125 ml
- Saltto taste
- Ground black pepperto taste

COOKING INSTRUCTION 25 MINUTES + 5 MINUTES

1. Tomatoes (you need very ripe, sweet) are cut into quarters, peeled from seeds - and in general it is better to cut out their whole wet core. Cut into small cubes and transfer to a bowl.

2. Trim large and strong olives on four sides, discard the core with the bone. Tear off leaves from basil branches, send to olive slices and thoroughly chop with a knife. Transfer everything to the tomatoes, add a tablespoon of olive oil, salt and pepper - and mix well.

3. Put a mozzarella ball in a jug or other high capacity, add whipping cream, salt, pepper and beat with a blender to a uniform state. If it turned out very thick, you can add more cream. Pour the mixture into a siphon and put it in the refrigerator for an hour.

4. Arrange the tomato tartare with olives and basil in martini glasses. Then a few croutons. However, croutons - this is already a voluntary matter, you can completely do without them.

5. Finally, fill the glasses with mozzarella and cream air cream using a siphon. For aroma, sprinkle with olive oil - quite a bit, a quarter teaspoon per serving. And serve immediately.

Grill marinade sauce

INGREDIENTS

- Soy sauce 2 tablespoons
- Red wine vinegar 1 teaspoon
- Cayenne pepperto taste
- Saltto taste
- Vegetable oil 2 tablespoons
- Ground black pepperto taste
- Garlic 1 clove

COOKING INSTRUCTION 20 MINUTES

1. Squeeze the garlic.

2. Add soy sauce, vinegar, vegetable oil, salt, pepper.

3. Knead until the salt dissolves.

Salted lemons

INGREDIENTS

- Lemon 1 kg
- Black peppercorns 1 teaspoon
- Bay leaf 3 pieces
- Salt 300 g
- Olive oil 150 ml

COOKING INSTRUCTION 10 MINUTES

1. Lemons (it is better to take not very large so that it is easier to put them in a jar) to wash, make cuts on them - as if we cut them into six parts, but do not cut them to the end.

2. From two cut lemons, first squeeze the juice with your hands in a liter jar, and then put all the lemons in it (squeezed including), add salt, pepper, bay leaf and pour all the olive oil.

3. Soak lemons for at least a month, and then they can be added to any unsweetened dishes, such as stews, and the oil itself can be added to salads.

Redcurrant Tkemali

INGREDIENTS

- Redcurrant 250 g
- Cilantro 70 g
- Coriander Seeds 10 g
- Caraway seeds 10 g
- Garlic 3 cloves
- Saltto taste

COOKING INSTRUCTION 20 MINUTES

1. In a mortar, mash coriander, caraway seeds, cilantro leaves and garlic until smooth.

2. Pour currants with water and boil for about five minutes.

3. Then rub through a sieve into a clean saucepan, add the mixture from the mortar and mix and put on the fire to boil until thickened.

Sun-dried tomato pesto

INGREDIENTS

- Sun-dried tomatoes 150 g
- Pine nuts 50 g
- Garlic 1 clove
- Basil 10 g
- Hard cheese70 g
- Olive oil 100 ml

COOKING INSTRUCTION 10 MINUTES

1. Grate the cheese, finely chop the basil.

2. In a blender, punch all the **INGREDIENTS** to a homogeneous consistency. If necessary, add some more olive oil.

3. Transfer the sauce to a clean, dry jar, and store in the refrigerator for no more than three weeks.

Chimichurri sauce

INGREDIENTS

- Parsley 100 g
- Cilantro 25 g
- Garlic 8 cloves
- Shallots 2 pieces
- Oregano 1 teaspoon
- Chili flakes 1 teaspoon
- Lemon 1 piece
- Red wine vinegar 60 ml
- Extra virgin olive oil 200 ml
- Saltto taste
- Ground black pepperto taste

COOKING INSTRUCTION 15 MINUTES

1. Grind parsley and cilantro, only leaves, stems are not needed.

2. At the cloves of garlic, remove the cores, they are bitter, and cut very finely. Finely chop the onion.

3. Combine herbs, garlic and onions in a bowl, add oregano, chili flakes, salt and pepper.

4. Add the juice of one lemon, vinegar, oil, mix well and let it brew for a couple of hours so that the tastes mix.

5. Serve the sauce to the steak. You can also store the sauce in a closed jar in the refrigerator for 1-2 weeks.

Plum and hot pepper sauce

INGREDIENTS
- Plums 300 g
- Chili pepper 1 piece
- Ground ½ teaspooncoriander
- Red basil 4 sprigs
- Sugar 2 tablespoons
- Wine vinegar1 tablespoon
- Port 4 tablespoons
- Water 1 cup

COOKING INSTRUCTION 40 MINUTES

1. Separate plum and capsicum from seeds and seeds.
2. Throw the plum into the stewpan and evaporate the port with it.
3. Then add water and add pepper, bring to a boil and reduce heat.
4. Add finely chopped basil, coriander, sugar and cook for another 10 minutes.
5. Add vinegar, salt and pepper to taste. Remove from heat and allow to cool to room temperature.
6. Beat the cooled plums with a blender and leave in the refrigerator overnight.

Cucumber Wright

INGREDIENTS
- Yogurt 560 g
- Cucumbers 250 g
- Cumin (Zira) 2 teaspoons
- Black mustard seeds 1 teaspoon
- Cilantro 20 g
- Saltto taste
- Ground black pepperto taste

COOKING INSTRUCTION 30 MINUTES

1. Slightly fry the cumin and black mustard in a dry frying pan, and then crush it in a mortar or using a processor.
2. Peel the cucumbers from the skin, remove the seeds (they give a lot of water) and cut into small cubes.
3. Beat yogurt thoroughly, add cucumbers, cumin and mustard, salt, pepper, add chopped cilantro and mix. Put in the refrigerator for the night. Serve with spicy Indian dishes.

Walnut adjika

INGREDIENTS
- Red Chilli 500 g
- Garlic 175 g
- Walnuts 75 g
- Utsho Suneli 25 g
- Salt1.5 teaspoons

COOKING INSTRUCTION 20 MINUTES

1. Peppers cut the stalk, leave the seeds, they will give sharpness.
2. Pass peppers, peeled garlic, and nuts through a meat grinder.
3. Add all the spices, mix well.

4. Squeeze the resulting mass through cheesecloth to get rid of excess juice. Transfer adjika to a jar and store in the refrigerator.

Matbuha

INGREDIENTS
- Red bell pepper 2 pieces
- Tomatoes 8 pieces
- Green chili pepper 1 piece
- Garlic 5 cloves
- Olive oil 80 ml
- Paprika 1 tablespoon
- Sugar 1 tablespoon
- Saltto taste
- Ground black pepperto taste

COOKING INSTRUCTION 2 HOURS

1. Grease red pepper with olive oil and put in the oven, preheated to 220 degrees, for 20 minutes. Pepper should become soft. Transfer hot pepper to a clean bowl, cover with foil and leave for 5 minutes. Remove the skin from it, remove the seeds and the stalk, cut the pulp into cubes with a side about a centimeter.

2. On tomatoes, make small cross-shaped incisions at both ends. Place them in boiling water for 30 seconds, then transfer them to ice water to stop cooking. Peel and chop the tomatoes in the same cubes as pepper.

3. Put prepared peppers and tomatoes, diced green peppers, chopped chili and garlic in a thick-walled pan. Put on medium heat and cook for 20 minutes, stirring occasionally.

4. Add oil, paprika, sugar, salt and pepper to vegetables. Cook, stirring constantly, for another 10 minutes. Then remove from heat and let cool. Serve matbuhu cold with pita.

Soaked plums

INGREDIENTS
- Plums 10 kg
- Water 5 L
- Sugar 200 g
- Salt 100 g
- Mustard Powder 30 g

COOKING INSTRUCTION 10 MINUTES

1. Mix water with sugar, salt and mustard powder.

2. Thoroughly wash the plums and pour them with brine. For flavor, you can add plum leaves.

3. After pouring the plums, cover the fruit surface with a cotton towel, put oppression on top. For 6-8 days, keep indoors at room temperature for pre-fermentation. Then put it in a cold place for a month. Plums can be used as a side dish for meat and fish dishes.

Pickled Beetroot Garlic

INGREDIENTS
- Garlic4 heads
- Water 500 ml
- Vinegar 9% 50 ml
- Salt 50 g
- Black pepper peas 10 pieces
- Allspice 2 peas
- Caraway seeds 1 teaspoon
- Bay leaf 1 piece
- Beetroot 50 g

COOKING INSTRUCTION 20 MINUTES + 15 DAYS

1. Remove the top husk from the garlic so that the heads remain intact, cut off the legs and cut off the roots.
2. Blanch the garlic in boiling water for 10 seconds, and then transfer to ice water to allow it to cool quickly.
3. Put the cooled garlic in a jar together with slices of fresh beets as tight as possible.
4. Boil water with salt and spices for the marinade, then remove from heat and add vinegar. Pour the garlic with hot marinade, close and let cool cool. Then put in the refrigerator. After 2 weeks, the garlic will be ready.

Thyrocafteri

INGREDIENTS
- 2 tablespoonsolive oil
- Feta cheese300 g
- Red wine vinegar2 tablespoons
- Chili pepper1 piece

COOKING INSTRUCTION 10 MINUTES

1. Remove the cuttings and seeds from the chili pepper and finely chop. In the presence of free time, pepper can be thrown into the oven for 5-20 minutes for a more expressive taste.
2. Put feta sliced into cubes in a bowl, add chili pepper, part of olive oil and beat with a blender to a homogeneous consistency.
3. Gradually add vinegar and the remaining olive oil into the cheese.

Mayonnaise pesto

INGREDIENTS
- Basil 15 g
- 2 tablespoonsolive oil
- Egg yolk 2 pieces
- Mustard 1 teaspoon
- Saltto taste
- White wine vinegar 1 teaspoon
- Vegetable oil 500 ml

COOKING INSTRUCTION 15 MINUTES

1. Lower the basil leaves for fifteen seconds in boiling water, pull out with a slotted spoon and transfer to ice water. Remove the basil, squeeze out the excess water - and put in a blender with two tablespoons of olive oil. Turn on the blender for about two minutes.
2. Beat in an emulsion two egg yolks, mustard and vinegar. Then gradually pour in the vegetable oil, constantly whipping the thickening mass until you get mayonnaise.
3. Stir a little water into the mayonnaise - depending on how thick the mayonnaise is, a different amount of liquid may be needed. The result should be a substance capable of pouring. Stir basil in it and add salt to taste.

Aioli

INGREDIENTS
- Garlic 1 head
- Olive oilto taste
- Saltpinch

COOKING INSTRUCTION 30 MINUTES

1. Peel the garlic and mash in a mortar with a pinch of salt until pasty or grate on a fine grater. Previously, from the garlic, get the core, cutting a clove in half.
2. Then pour in a thin stream of olive oil (it is not necessary to use extra virgin oil here, olive oil is better for softer) and continuously whisk with a whisk in one direction. Throughout the preparation of the sauce, do not change the direction of movement of the whisk.
3. The sauce is ready when it is thick enough to stand a spoon in it.

Sandwich Recipes

Grilled Beef, Ham and Cheese Sandwiches

INGREDIENTS

- Mustard 6 tablespoons
- French baguette 1 piece
- Beef tenderloin 140 g
- Ham 140 g
- Pickled Cucumbers 0.3 cups
- Provolone cheese 140 g
- Butter 2 tablespoons
- Saltto taste
- Vegetable oilto taste
- Ground black pepperto taste

COOKING INSTRUCTION 30 MINUTES

1. Preheat the grill or barbecue. Lubricate the meat with vegetable oil, salt and pepper. Put on the grill and fry for several minutes, turning until tender. Cool slightly and chop finely.
2. Cut the baguette across in half, then each half along in half, without cutting to the end. Lubricate the bread with mustard on the inside, put the thinly sliced meat, thinly sliced ham, thinly sliced cheese and thinly sliced cucumbers. Cover the sandwiches and coat the outside with softened butter.
3. Put in the grill for grill, close and fry on both sides for 2-3 minutes. Cut each sandwich in half and serve immediately.

Chicken and Bacon Sandwiches

INGREDIENTS

- Bacon 100 g
- Chicken fillet 300 g
- Green salad 1 bunch
- Tomatoes 1 piece
- Cucumbers 1 g
- Sweet red onion 1 piece
- Mustardto taste
- Toast bread 300 g
- Cheese 100 g

COOKING INSTRUCTION 30 MINUTES

1. Cut the chicken fillet into thin plates and fry in oil with spices.
2. Tomato, cucumber and onion cut into rings.
3. Cheese cut into triangular plates in the calculation of 2 triangles per 1 sandwich.
4. Heat the bread in a toaster and coat with sauce (mustard).
5. Put lettuce on the toast, then vegetables, chicken and cheese.
6. Fry the slices of bacon and put in a sandwich immediately before serving. Cover with a second toast.

Crab Meat Sandwich

INGREDIENTS

- Ciabatta 1 piece
- Cream Cheese 30 g
- Grana padano cheese 100 g
- Edam cheese 100 g
- A mixture of lettuce leaves 1 bunch
- Tomatoes 1 piece
- Crab meat 100 g

COOKING INSTRUCTION 10 MINUTES PRINT
1. Cut the ciabatta in half. Spread with melted cheese.
2. Put 2 slices of cheese.
3. Cut or split crab meat by hand. Put on cheese.
4. Put lettuce leaves and two slices of tomato on top.
5. Pepper. You can add a drop of olive oil.
6. Close the sandwich.
7. Cut in half.

Quick salmon, vegetable and ricotta sandwiches

INGREDIENTS
- Canned Salmon 400 g
- Red onion 60 g
- Extra virgin olive oil 1 tablespoon
- Lemon juice 2 tablespoons
- Freshly ground black pepperto taste
- Pumpernickel 8 pieces
- 4 tablespoonsricotta cheese
- Tomatoes 8 pieces
- Lettuce leaves 2 pieces

COOKING INSTRUCTION 30 MINUTES
1. In a bowl, mix the fish, chopping into pieces, finely chopped onions, lemon juice, olive oil and a little black pepper.
2. Spread the cheese on 4 slices of bread and put the fish mass, slices of tomatoes and slices of lettuce on top.
3. Cover with the remaining bread, gently squeeze and cut each sandwich in half diagonally.

Camembert and Fig Morning Sandwich

INGREDIENTS
- Ciabatta 1 piece
- Figs 2 pieces
- Camembert cheese 50 g
- Walnuts 3 tablespoons
- Honey 2 tablespoons
- Olive oilto taste
- Green saladto taste

COOKING INSTRUCTION 10 MINUTES
1. Cut the ciabatta in half across, and then in half lengthwise. Fry the bread, crust up, in a pan in a small amount of butter until golden brown.
2. Mix nuts and honey. Put lettuce, cheese, chopped figs on a slightly cooled bread and nut-honey mixture on top.

Soft Cheese Sandwiches

INGREDIENTS
- Ricotta cheese 100 g
- Mascarpone cheese 100 g
- Cream 40% 2 tablespoons
- Chives 1 bunch
- White bread 10 slices
- Rye bread 10 slices

COOKING INSTRUCTION 30 MINUTES
1. Chop the onion finely. Combine both cheeses, then add cream and a tablespoon of chopped onion.

2. Cut the crusts from the bread, spread the cheese mixture into slices of wheat bread and cover with rye bread.

3. Cut each sandwich diagonally to make triangles. You can serve immediately, but you can first hold a little in the refrigerator.

Tuna and fried egg sandwich

INGREDIENTS
- Canned tuna in own juice 70 g
- Ciabatta 1 piece
- Quail egg 5 pieces
- Arugula 10 g
- Butter 1 teaspoon
- Mayonnaise 1 tablespoon

COOKING INSTRUCTION 15 MINUTES

1. Cut the ciabatta into two parts.

2. Mash tuna with a fork and mix well with mayonnaise.

3. Put tuna on both halves of the ciabatta.

4. Meanwhile, prepare the scrambled eggs so that the yolks remain liquid.

5. On one half put the fried eggs, on top of the arugula, close the second half of the ciabatta.

6. When serving, cut into 4 parts.

Sandwich with Tuna, Artichokes and Paprika

INGREDIENTS
- Ciabatta 2 pieces
- Garlic 4 heads
- Green basil 1 bunch
- Canned tuna in own juice 3 cans
- Kalamata olives 20 pieces
- Red bell pepper 2 pieces
- Red onion 1 head
- Chopped parsleyto taste
- Artichokes in oil 1 can
- Lemon juice 3 tablespoons
- Olive oil 3 tablespoons
- Saltto taste
- Ground black pepperto taste

COOKING INSTRUCTION 45 MINUTES

1. Cut the ciabatta lengthwise into two parts. Cut a little crumb from the middle so that there is more room for filling. You can fry a little bread in a grill pan on both sides. Grease with olive oil and grate with garlic, lay out basil leaves.

2. Mix finely chopped tuna, olives, bell pepper, red onion, artichokes and parsley.

3. Prepare the dressing: beat with a whisk olive oil and lemon juice to get a thick cloudy emulsion. Fill the resulting sauce with a mixture of tuna and vegetables.

4. Put the mixture in ciabatta, squeeze the halves of the bread properly, wrap it in baking paper and take it with you to a picnic or to work!

Fried Shrimp Sandwich

INGREDIENTS
- Peeled Shrimp 450 g
- Kacup cornmeal
- Wheat flour ¾ cup
- Kajun spices 3 tablespoons
- Salt1 teaspoon

- Chicken egg 2 pieces
- Peanut Butter 150 g
- Lett ½ bunch
- Tomatoes 2 g
- Pikuli 2 pieces
- Creole mustard 2.5 tablespoons
- Small French baguette 4 pieces
- Mayonnaise 240 g
- Tabasco red sauce 1 teaspoon
- Marinade 1 tablespoon
- Sweet paprika 1 tablespoon

COOKING INSTRUCTION 15 MINUTES

1. Mix the **INGREDIENTS** for the remoulade sauce: mustard, mayonnaise, marinade, tabasco, paprika, 2 tablespoons of the Khajun mixture - and set aside.
2. Pour enough oil on a large frying pan (or wok) and heat. Combine the corn and wheat flour, the remaining kajun mixture and salt in a bowl. Beat eggs slightly, dip the shrimp first in the egg mixture, and then quickly roll in the flour. Spread the shrimp in razoretnoy butter and fry until golden brown. Put the shrimp on a napkin so that it absorbs excess fat.
3. Cut mini-baguettes along, grease each half with remoulade. On the lower parts put circles of pickles, lettuce, tomatoes, and then fried shrimp. Cover the sandwiches with the upper halves and squeeze lightly.
4. Serve with sauce and beer.

Norwegian herring sandwich

INGREDIENTS
- Norwegian slightly salted herring1 piece
- Sour cream 100 g
- Gherkins 4 pieces
- A mixture of lettuce leaves 100 g
- Red bell pepper 50 g
- Wine Vinegar 20 ml
- Olive oil 70 ml
- Chives 2 stalks
- Parsley 1 bunch
- Rye bread 200 g

COOKING INSTRUCTION 15 MINUTES

1. Cut the Norwegian herring into fillets and cut into slices. Grease brown bread with sour cream, put salad leaves, slices of herring and gherkins on it. Sprinkle with a mixture of vinegar and olive oil.
2. Garnish sandwiches with a long straw of sweet pepper, sprinkle with chopped green onions and parsley.

Sandwich with tongue, arugula and champignons

INGREDIENTS
- Armenian lavash 1 piece
- Tomatoes flame 1 piece
- Arugula 1 bunch
- Fresh champignons 4 pieces
- Truffle oil 1 teaspoon
- 2 tablespoonsolive oil
- Dried thymeto taste
- Ground black pepperto taste
- Saltto taste

- Veal tongue 100 g

COOKING INSTRUCTION 15 MINUTES

1. Cut the tongue into thin long slices and fry in olive oil, salt, pepper and add thyme to taste.
2. Lightly fry the champignons in olive oil, put in a clean bowl, trying to leave excess oil in a pan. Drizzle with truffle oil to give the mushrooms a flavor.
3. Put the arugula, thin slices of tomato, mushrooms and tongue evenly on the unfolded pita bread.
4. Wrap tightly, if necessary, cut off excess pita bread along the edges. Cut into two and serve.

Sandwiches Mozzarella in Carozza

INGREDIENTS
- White bread for toast 12 slices
- Milk 200 ml
- Wheat flour 160 g
- Mozzarella Cheese 300 g
- Extra virgin olive oil 100 ml
- Chicken egg 3 pieces
- Saltto taste

COOKING INSTRUCTION 20 MINUTES

1. In one plate, beat eggs lightly, salt. Pour flour into the second. Pour milk into the third.
2. Cut mozzarella 1 cm thick.
3. Heat the oil in a pan.
4. Quickly dip two pieces of bread (without crust) in milk, put 2 pieces of mozzarella on one, and squeeze a second piece of bread.
5. Then roll in flour, then in egg and send to a hot pan, fry over high heat for 1.5 minutes on each side (at the same time, fry no more than two sandwiches so that they do not stick together). Serve right away.

English cucumber sandwiches

INGREDIENTS
- Butter 2 tablespoons
- Fresh mint 2 stalks
- Whole Grain Bread 6 Slices
- Cream Cheese 2 Tbsp
- Cucumbers 1 piece
- Saltto taste

COOKING INSTRUCTION 10 MINUTES

1. Wash, dry, mint, peel and finely chop.
2. Mix well with butter and cheese.
3. Brush the resulting mixture with pieces of bread.
4. Wash the cucumber, cut into very thin circles.
5. Arrange the mugs in 3 pieces of bread.
6. Lightly salt and cover with the remaining bread.
7. Cut off the peel sandwiches and cut each diagonally into 4 parts.

Sandwiches with Autumn Vegetables

INGREDIENTS
- Zucchini 2 pieces
- Eggplant 1 piece
- Tomatoes 3 pieces
- Onion 1 head
- Carrot 1 piece
- Sugarto taste
- Tomato paste 3 tablespoons

- Saltto taste
- Ground black pepperto taste
- 2 tablespoonsolive oil
- 1 piececheese
- Rustic bread 2 slices
- Dried basilto taste

COOKING INSTRUCTION 1 HOUR 10 MINUTES + 5 MINUTES

1. Vegetables must be washed thoroughly. Cut the eggplant into circles (thickness greater than .5 cm, but less than 1 cm). Dip in salty cold water.

2. Peel the zucchini and cut into rings of approximately the same thickness as the eggplant. If zucchini is young, then the core can not be cut, but if it is mature or a specific variety with large seeds, then the flesh is carefully cut (cutting the pentagon with a knife in circles is the easiest way). Spread the rings on a plate and sprinkle with salt.

3. Tomatoes cut across the rings as thick as eggplant. Cut a few circles into cubes, set aside the rest.

4. Grate the carrots on a coarse grater and cut the onion into cubes. In a heated frying pan, spasser the carrots, onions and tomato cubes for 10 minutes.

5. Turn on the oven 200 degrees. Dilute the tomato paste with a small amount of water (so that it looks like a very thick tomato juice), salt, pepper, add sugar. Pour the carrot sauce with onions and tomatoes and mix. This mixture will flavored vegetables.

6. Put vegetables in a heat-resistant form: a layer of zucchini slices, a layer of eggplant slices, then a teaspoon of sauce for each column, zucchini, tomatoes, sauce again ... Sprinkle with freshly ground pepper, cover with foil and put in the oven. After 50 minutes, the vegetable appetizer and filling are ready.

7. Fry slices of bread in a toaster. Put a portion of vegetables on one half, sprinkle with basil rubbed in the palms, then a slice of cheese - and cover with the second half of bread. If the column of vegetables is too high, then you can divide it by 2. We put it in the microwave for 30 seconds.

Low Calorie Tuna Sandwich

INGREDIENTS
- Rye bun 1 piece
- Curd cheese 40 g
- Canned tuna in own juice 50 g
- Red onion 2 pieces
- Tomatoes 2 pieces
- Chicken egg 1 piece
- Mix of lettuce leaves Tango mix "Belaya Dacha"1 bunch
- Balsamic vinegarto taste

COOKING INSTRUCTION 15 MINUTES

1. Cut the bun in half

2. Spread cottage cheese with cheese, put tuna, put onion rings, tomato slices and finely chopped boiled egg, add salad mix and pour balsamic vinegar.

3. Cover with the second half of the rolls.

Light prosciutto and mozzarella sandwiches

INGREDIENTS
Prosciutto 2 pieces
Canned fried peppers 2 pieces
Mozzarella Cheese 90 g
Whole grain bread 4 pieces

COOKING INSTRUCTION 30 MINUTES

1. Put prosciutto, slices of cheese and chopped peppers on 2 slices of bread. Top with the remaining bread and gently squeeze. Cut each in half diagonally.

Grilled Chicken Sandwiches with BBQ Sauce

INGREDIENTS

- Grilled chicken 1.2 kg
- Barbecue sauce 1.5 cups
- ½ cuppineapple jam
- Chili powder 1 teaspoon
- 24 piecebread toast
- Lettuce 1 piece
- Tomatoes 2 pieces

COOKING INSTRUCTION 15 MINUTES

1. Remove the skin from the chicken. Separate the meat from the bones and cut into small pieces. Cut the tomatoes into slices and get rid of seeds and excess fluid.

2. In a pan, combine barbecue sauce, jam and chili. Put on medium heat, add chicken and cook, stirring, for about 5 minutes.

Goat Cheese and Spinach Sandwich

INGREDIENTS

- White bread 1 piece
- Butterto taste
- Goat cheese 70 g
- Canned Peppers 2 pieces
- Spinach 30 g

COOKING INSTRUCTION 5 MINUTES

1. Cut the bread into large pieces, spread them with butter and put the butter up on the board.

2. Put goat cheese, peppers and spinach on one piece of bread. Cover with another piece of bread, press firmly. Trim the crusts, cut diagonally into triangles and serve.

Sandwiches with Parma ham, Gallic melon and green basil

INGREDIENTS

- Ciabatta 6 pieces
- Parma ham2 00 g
- Gallic melon 1 piece
- Olive oil 50 ml
- Green basil 1 bunch
- Lemon 1 piece
- Ground black pepperto taste

COOKING INSTRUCTION 5 MINUTES

1. Six small ciabatta loaves cut in half. Grease each half with a sauce consisting of extra virgin olive oil, lemon juice and black pepper. As an aromatic bonus, you can put a little Modena balsamic in the sauce, but, in principle, this is not necessary.

2. On bread, put Parma ham cut in the thinnest slices, sliced thicker sliced sugar Gallic melon, put on each sandwich two lush branches of green basil and cover the top with the second half of ciabatta. There are hands, washed down with bubbly, slightly sweet wine Lambrusco.

Sandwich with Chicken and Vegetables

INGREDIENTS

- Onion 1 piece
- Cucumbers 3 pieces
- ½ cuptable vinegar
- Mayonnaise 10 tablespoons
- 16 piece bread toast
- Chicken breast fillet 3 pieces

COOKING INSTRUCTION 1 HOUR + 5 MINUTES

1. Cut the onion into small half rings and soak in a mixture of vinegar and water (half a glass of vinegar and half a glass of water). Leave it overnight.

2. Cut the chicken breast into small pieces and fry until tender (if you want a diet sandwich, boil or grill). Cool and cut into thin slices. Cut the cucumbers into thin slices. Remove the onion from the marinade and let the excess liquid drain.

3. Lubricate the bread with mayonnaise on one side (for diet - low-calorie sour cream with finely chopped herbs). Lay on top slices of cucumber, slices of chicken, onions, top slice of bread. Press with your palms so that the sandwich does not fall apart, cut into portions and serve.

Sandwiches with celery salad and remoulade sauce

INGREDIENTS
- Celery Root 200 g
- Crab Meat 50 g
- Egg yolk 2 pieces
- Sugar ½ teaspoon
- Vegetable oil 200 ml
- Salt 4 g
- Vinegar 1 tablespoon
- Mustard 1 tablespoon
- Lemon juice 30 ml
- Gherkins 20 g
- Capers 20 g
- Tarragonto taste
- Green apples ¼ pieces
- Lettuce leaves 4 pieces
- French baguette 2 pieces

COOKING INSTRUCTION 15 MINUTES

1. For remoulade you will need homemade mayonnaise: beat yolks with salt, sugar and mustard in a mixer; after a minute, continuing to whisk, pour vegetable oil in a thin stream, and after it - vinegar and a tablespoon of water.

2. Add finely chopped gherkins and capers to the mayonnaise, as well as chopped tarragon, pour in the lemon juice and mix well.

3. Peel half the celery root and grate on a medium grater. Do the same with a peeled quarter of a green apple. Coarsely chop the crab meat. Transfer everything to a bowl, season with remoulade and mix.

4. Cut not too long baguettes in half, and half lengthwise. Put the salad on all eight pieces, smooth it out - and combine the halves of the sandwiches, putting in the middle of the lettuce leaf.

Fried Egg, Bacon and Cheese Sandwich

INGREDIENTS
- Bacon 10 g
- White bread ½ pieces
- Edam cheese 20 g
- Tomatoes 1 piece
- Mayonnaise 1 tablespoon
- Butter 10 g
- Chicken egg 1 piece
- Lettuce leaves 3 pieces

COOKING INSTRUCTION 5 MINUTES

1. Fry thin slices of bacon until golden brown.

2. Heat the bread and spread one half of the sandwich with mayonnaise (you can make it yourself), put cheese, tomato slices, bacon and lettuce on the second.

3. Meanwhile, in butter, fry a little fried eggs - such that the yolk is half-cooked.

Sandwiches with Tuna and Cheese

INGREDIENTS
- Canned tuna in own juice 1 can
- Bread for toasts 8 slices
- Emmental cheese 200 g
- Pink pepperto taste
- Capers ½ teaspoon
- Butter 20 g
- Cucumbers ½ pieces

COOKING INSTRUCTION 10 MINUTES

1. Put the tuna together with the juice in a bowl and knead it with your hands. Sprinkle with pink Mauritius pepper (it is as fragrant as black, but less hot), add capers and mix. Put grated emmental (or other cheese to taste - edam, for example, or gouda) and mix again.

2. Heat the pan over medium heat and lightly dry the bread on both sides. Then lightly grease all the pieces on one side with butter, put the tuna-cheese mixture, combine the halves of the sandwiches - and again send to the skillet. There they should spend a couple of minutes under the lid - the idea is to melt the cheese and grab the fish mass.

Tuna sandwich

INGREDIENTS
- Canned tuna in its own juice 2 cans
- Light mayonnaise ¼ g
- Granular mustard 2 tablespoons
- Chives 1 bunch
- Sweet red onion 1 head
- Celery 1 stalk
- Green apples 1 piece
- Cucumbers 1 piece
- Chicken egg (large) 2 pieces
- Green saladto taste

COOKING INSTRUCTION 20 MINUTES

1. Any bread you like: ciabatta, baguette, black, Borodino. It's best to fry it a little without oil or make toasts (we use toasts).

2. Drain the tuna, chop finely and mix all the **INGREDIENTS**.

3. Put on a toast decorated with a leaf of salad, cover with a second piece of bread.

Bacon Club Sandwich

INGREDIENTS
- Bacon 400 g
- Meat 8 pieces
- 4 piececheese
- Red onion 1 piece
- Mayonnaise 100 g
- White bread 8 slices
- Tomatoes 8 pieces
- Green salad 4 pieces

COOKING INSTRUCTION 10 MINUTES

1. In a pan, fry slices of bread on one side. On the non-roasted side, we smear the mayonnaise.

2. Put cheese and bacon on top, then meat.

3. Then two slices of tomato, chopped onion, lettuce.

Sandwiches with salmon and Rondele cheese

INGREDIENTS
- Rondele cheese 95 g
- Olive oil 2 teaspoons
- White bread 8 slices
- Balsamic vinegar 2 teaspoons
- Dill 8 stems
- Lightly salted salmon 4 pieces
- Lettuce leaves 4 pieces
- Ground black pepperto taste

COOKING INSTRUCTION 5 MINUTES

1. Put the cheese in a bowl, add olive oil and balsamic vinegar, mix. Pepper to taste, add finely chopped tops of four branches of dill, mix again.
2. Put four slices of bread on a sheet of lettuce, spread on top with cheese. Spread the remaining bread with cheese.
3. Put a slice of salmon on bread with lettuce and cover with the remaining pieces of bread. Top with a sprig of dill.

Herring sandwich

INGREDIENTS
- Bun 3 pieces
- Herring fillet 6 pieces
- ½ sweet onion
- Pickled cucumbers 3 pieces

COOKING INSTRUCTION 5 MINUTES

1. Finely chop the onion. Cut the cucumbers into thin slices.
2. Cut herring fillets into small pieces.
3. Put herring fillet on both sides of the bun - top and bottom. Sprinkle with onion and cover with cucumber.

Chicken and Tomato Sandwich

INGREDIENTS
- 2 toast bread
- Chicken fillet 1 piece
- Gouda cheese 1 piece
- Buko cheese 30 g
- Tomatoes 1 piece
- Green salad 1 bunch

COOKING INSTRUCTION 10 MINUTES

1. Boil chicken fillet. Cut lengthwise 1-2 cm.
2. Spread bread with cheese buko.
3. On the lower bread, put gouda cheese and a slice of chicken.
4. On the top - salad leaf and a slice of tomato.
5. Connect the sandwich.

Smoked Salmon Avocado Sandwiches

INGREDIENTS
- Avocado 1 piece
- Light mayonnaise 1 tablespoon
- ½ teaspoonlemon juice
- Freshly ground black pepperto taste
- 8whole grain bread

- Smoked Salmon 60 g
- Cucumbers 1 piece

COOKING INSTRUCTION 30 MINUTES

1. Peel and cut avocados into thin slices. Cut the cucumber into thin circles.
2. In a small bowl, combine mayonnaise, lemon juice, and a little black pepper.
3. Spread the bread with the sauce. Half the avocado slices, thinly sliced fish and cucumber. Top with the remaining bread and gently squeeze. Cut each in half diagonally.

Turkey, Cheese and Arugula Sandwich

INGREDIENTS
- Rye bread 2 slices
- Turkey fillet 50 g
- Tomatoes 2 pieces
- Arugulato taste
- Emmental cheese 20 g

COOKING INSTRUCTION 30 MINUTES

1. Boil the turkey fillet.
2. Put the fillet on the bottom bread, on top - a slice of tomato and cover everything with a slice of cheese.
3. Turn the top bread, put a second slice of cheese and tomato.
4. Send the buter to the microwave for 30 seconds.
5. Between the buters put arugula or some other greenery and connect the two halves.

Sandwich with Bacon, Cheese and Fresh Vegetables

INGREDIENTS
- Mustard 10 g
- Mayonnaise 10 g
- Tomatoes 20 g
- Cucumbers 20 g
- Green salad 20 g
- Onion 20 g
- Bacon 2 slices
- 2 piececheese
- Chopped bread 2 pieces

COOKING INSTRUCTION 15 MINUTES

1. Spread one slice of bread with mayonnaise, the other with mustard.
2. Fry the bacon and put it on the bread with mustard.
3. Cut into slices tomatoes, cucumbers, onions. Put onions on bacon, then - tomato, cucumber and salad. Cut the cheese and put on a piece of bread, spread with mayonnaise.
4. Fold together and slice diagonally.

Fried egg sandwich

INGREDIENTS
- Olive oilto taste
- French baguette 1 piece
- Butter 50 g
- 4 eggs
- Tomato pasteto taste
- Saltto taste
- Ground black pepperto taste

COOKING INSTRUCTION 30 MINUTES

1. Cut the loaf along, but not to the end (as if it were a big sandwich). Preheat the grill pan. Sprinkle the bread with butter from the inside, rub and squeeze the butter side down on the grill pan.

2. At this time, heat a large frying pan over medium heat, add half the cubes of oil. Let them melt and start foaming. Gently break the eggs into the pan without damaging the yolk. Protein lightly salt. Fry the eggs for 3-4 minutes, until the yolks settle slightly, add the remaining half of the oil in the process.

3. Using a spatula with holes, remove the fried eggs from the pan, drain the oil, put on one of the toasted sides of the bread. Pepper and add tomato paste. Cover with the second half of bread, cut in half. Eat right away.

Banana sandwich

INGREDIENTS
- Bananas 2 pieces
- White bread 4 slices
- Chicken egg 1 piece
- ½ cupmilk
- Ground cinnamon ½ tablespoon
- Saltpinch
- Butter 1 tablespoon
- Maple syrupto taste
- Powdered sugarto taste

COOKING INSTRUCTION 15 MINUTES

1. Beat with whisk cinnamon, salt, eggs, milk
2. Put slices of bread in a bowl for impregnation.
3. Fry bread to a skillet, to melted butter
4. Turn over, put half the banana.
5. Cover with another slice and press firmly.
6. Fry on all sides.
7. Sprinkle with honey or maple syrup, sprinkle with powdered sugar, if desired.

Cheese and fish club sandwich

INGREDIENTS
- Cheese "Lambert" 50% fat 50 g
- White bread 4 slices
- Smoked trout 50 g
- Green salad 50 g
- Tomatoes10 g
- Chives 5 g
- Cucumbers 10 g
- Yogurt 50 g
- Anchovies 10 g
- Garlic 2 cloves

COOKING INSTRUCTION 20 MINUTES

1. Bake the grilled bread on both sides.
2. Tomato, cucumber, cheese and trout cut into thin slices.
3. Mash anchovies in a mortar with garlic, add yogurt, seboulet and mix.
4. Grease the toasts on one side with yogurt sauce.
5. Put the lettuce, tomato, cucumber, cheese, fish on the first toast.
6. Cover with a second slice of fried bread, repeat the layers and cover with a third.
7. Trim the peels and serve.

Sandwich with Bacon, Salad and Tomatoes

INGREDIENTS
- White bread 2 slices
- Bacon 2 pieces
- Mayonnaise 3 tablespoons

- Tomatoes 3 pieces
- Romano salad 2 pieces

COOKING INSTRUCTION 20 MINUTES

1. Fry the bread in a toaster, in no case bringing it to a cracker condition.

2. In mayonnaise (it is best to make homemade), add a little olive oil, squeeze the garlic in it and drip Tabasco or freshly ground pepper.

3. To achieve beautiful, crispy slices, spread the bacon on a cold baking sheet, place in a cold oven and start heating it to 200'C. After 15-20 minutes, the bacon will acquire a characteristic crunch and color - the main thing is not to overdry. Put the bacon immediately on a paper towel to absorb excess fat.

4. Cut the tomatoes in circles half a centimeter thick.

5. Fold lettuce according to the size of the slices of bread.

6. Put the **INGREDIENTS** together, place on a large preheated plate.

Cold Chicken Sandwiches

INGREDIENTS

- Chicken breast fillet 2 pieces
- Soy sauce 2 tablespoons
- Rice vinegar 1 tablespoon
- Ground dried garlic ½ teaspoon
- Peppers mixto taste

COOKING INSTRUCTION 1 HOUR + 1 HOUR

1. Each fillet cut into 2 parts and beat off slightly. Put in a pan, add sauce, vinegar and garlic. Mix with your hands and let the chicken marinate in the refrigerator for an hour

2. Preheat the oven - "grill with convection" to 200 degrees.

3. Put breasts on a double layer of foil 4 pcs. beside. Sprinkle with freshly ground pepper. Wrap in a foil envelope and send to the oven. If the chicken gave juice, then you can pour them breasts before baking.

4. Leave in the oven for 30 minutes, 5 minutes before the end - open the flaps of the envelope so that a golden crust appears.

5. Refrigerate without removing from foil and put in the refrigerator.

Grilled cheese and apple sandwiches

INGREDIENTS

- Green apples 1 piece
- Whole grain bread 250 g
- Cheddar Cheese 240 g
- Olive oilto taste

COOKING INSTRUCTION 30 MINUTES

1. Preheat the grill or barbecue.

2. Cut the cheese into 8 thin slices. Thinly chop the apple. Put 4 slices of bread on the working surface, put a piece of cheese on each, then a layer of apples, then a layer of cheese and cover with the remaining bread. Sprinkle olive oil on both sides and grill.

3. Fry for about 5 minutes, turning over 1 time, until the sandwiches are browned and the cheese is melted. Lay on a board and cut in half.

Omelette Sandwiches

INGREDIENTS

- White bread for toast 8 slices
- Ham 200 g
- Green salad 1 bunch
- 4 eggs
- Tomatoes 1 piece
- Saltpinch
- Ground black pepperon the tip of a knife
- Mayonnaise 50 g

- Sliced cream cheese 4 pieces
- Butter 1 teaspoon

COOKING INSTRUCTION 15 MINUTES

1. On a dish on which you will serve sandwiches, put 4 slices of toaster bread and grease with mayonnaise.
2. Top with ham on each toast.
3. Then cut the tomato into thin circles and lay the ham on top.
4. Wash and dry lettuce sheets with paper towels and lay on top of the tomato.
5. In a glass, beat eggs, add salt, pepper and beat well with a fork.
6. Heat the pan, melt the butter and pour in the mixture with eggs and cover.
7. Divide the finished omelet into 4 equal parts with a wooden spatula and put hot on a lettuce leaf.
8. Place cheese on top of the omelet, cover each sandwich with toast and squeeze well.
9. Cut obliquely.

White bread sandwiches with mincemeat and apple

INGREDIENTS
- Herring fillet 300 g
- Chicken egg 2 pieces
- Green apples ¾ pieces
- Butter 70 g
- Ground black pepperto taste
- White bread for toast 2 slices

COOKING INSTRUCTION 15 MINUTES

1. The main ingredient of foreshmak is herring. If you buy a whole, then you need to soak it in milk (maybe an hour, or better - all night), and then rinse thoroughly: it will become more tender. Fillet, which is sold already packed, can not be soaked, but immediately passed through a meat grinder along with hard-boiled eggs and half a green apple peeled and peeled ("grenni smith" or something similar). Then add the butter sliced in medium cubes, mix and again pass through a meat grinder. At any of these stages, add ground pepper.
2. Dry the pieces of bread in a pan. Quarter the apple to get rid of the seeds (the remaining quarter can be eaten just like that) and cut into thin slices.
3. Spread all pieces of bread with an equal amount of forcemeat. Put apple slices in four pieces on top of the mincemeat. Combine half the sandwiches, and whole - cut diagonally.

Smoked Mozzarella Sandwiches

INGREDIENTS
- Ciabatta 8 pieces
- Butterto taste
- Smoked Mozzarella Cheese 12 pieces
- Tomatoes 2 pieces
- Basil leaves 8 pieces

COOKING INSTRUCTION 30 MINUTES

1. Remove from heat and cut each sandwich into 3 pieces. Arrange in 4 plates and serve hot, sprinkled with sea salt.
2. Preheat the grill. Spread each piece of bread with butter. Put 4 slices on a plate, butter side down, put cheese, chopped tomato and a basil leaf on top. Top with the remaining bread, butter side up.
3. Place the sandwiches on the grill, pressing lightly.
4. Fry for 3 minutes, pressing while cooking, turn over and fry for another 2 minutes, pressing again. Fry until the bread is browned and the filling melts.

Sprat Sandwiches

INGREDIENTS
- French baguette 1 piece
- Garlic 4 cloves
- Mayonnaise 250 g
- Ground black pepperto taste
- Sprats 1 can
- Cucumbers 1 piece

COOKING INSTRUCTION 20 MINUTES

1. Cut a long French loaf, fry each slice, set aside.
2. On one can of mayonnaise add 3-4 cloves of chopped garlic, a pinch of ground black pepper and beat.
3. On a fried slice of a loaf with a thick layer, smear the mayonnaise mass, put one sprat on top, decorate with greens, fresh cucumber.

Tuna and Avocado Sandwich

INGREDIENTS
- Avocado 1 piece
- Canned Tuna 1 can
- White bread for toast 6 slices
- Tomatoes 1 piece
- Sea saltat the tip of a knife
- Iceberg Salad 6 pieces
- Freshly ground black pepperon the tip of a knife
- Parsley 6 stems
- Lemon juice 1 tablespoon
- Sweet red onion 1 head

COOKING INSTRUCTION 10 MINUTES

1. Dry the bread in the toaster. Cut in half with a triangle.
2. Peel the avocado from the skin, remove the stone, crush or scroll to a puree state.
3. Finely chop the parsley, add to the avocado along with salt, pepper and lemon juice, stir.
4. Put salad, tomato slices, onion rings and mashed avocado on one half of each toast. Mash a little tuna with a fork, put on top. Cover with the second half of the toast.

Salmon and Avocado Sandwich

INGREDIENTS
- French baguette 1 piece
- Lightly salted salmon 100 g
- Avocado 1 piece

COOKING INSTRUCTION 10 MINUTES

1. Avocado and salmon cut into thin slices.
2. Put the avocado and salmon inside the baguette.
3. Avocado in this case is intended to replace ordinary butter. Very tasty.
4. Cut the baguette to the side, but not to the end.

Chopping Club Sandwich

INGREDIENTS
- Bacon 300 g
- Carbonade 250 g
- Cheese 150 g
- Red onion 1 piece
- Mayonnaiseto taste
- 6 toast bread

- Tomatoes 1 piece
- Green salad 300 g

COOKING INSTRUCTION 20 MINUTES

1. Dry the bread in a toaster, fry the bacon in a pan on both sides.
2. Spread one side of bread with a little mayonnaise, put in carbonate, bacon (the bigger, the tastier), cheese, 2 slices of tomato, chopped onion (optional) and salad (put all the products in this order).
3. Cover with a second piece of bread, and cut diagonally.

Club sandwich

INGREDIENTS
- 12 piece bread toast
- Mayonnaise 145 g
- Dijon mustard 30 g
- Lettuce leaves 8 pieces
- Cheddar Cheese 8 slices
- Turkey Breast 500 g
- Tomatoes 1 piece
- Bacon8 pieces

COOKING INSTRUCTION 15 MINUTES

1. Fry the bread in a toaster or oven until golden brown.
2. Fry the bacon in a frying pan without oil until golden brown.
3. Mix 85 grams of mayonnaise and Dijon mustard, grease with this sauce one side of each piece of bread, using about one teaspoon of sauce per piece.
4. Build a sandwich: put a lettuce leaf on the bottom toast, then a piece of cheese, a couple of slices of turkey, tomato rings, cover with the second toast with the sauce down, grease it with a teaspoon of mayonnaise, put another piece of cheese, a couple of slices of turkey, bacon, salad on top, cover third toast. Stick two skewers into the sandwich so that it does not fall apart, and cut it diagonally.

Chicken Club Sandwich

INGREDIENTS
- Chicken Breast 300 g
- 6 toast bread
- Tomatoes 2 pieces
- Mayonnaise 100 g
- Soy sauce 20 ml
- Turmeric 8 g
- Garlic 4 cloves
- Freshly ground black pepperto taste
- Cheese 150 g
- Green saladto taste

COOKING INSTRUCTION 30 MINUTES PRINT

1. Put the chicken breasts to cook.
2. Make the sauce. Mix mayonnaise with crushed garlic, soy sauce and turmeric. Add black pepper to taste.
3. Cut the sandwich bread into two triangular pieces. Spread one part with sauce
4. Finely and finely chop the chicken breast and put on top on the bread spread with the sauce.
5. Cut the cheese into 2 parts, put the cheese on the breast.
6. Peel the tomato from the skin, cut into thin (!!!) round slices, put on top
7. Grease the sauce again
8. Put the lettuce leaf
9. Cover with a second triangular slice

Sandwich "Gondolier"

INGREDIENTS

- Wheat bun 1 piece
- Cucumbers 30 g
- Tomatoes 30 g
- Red onion 30 g
- Green peas 30 g
- Ham 30 g
- Garlic 2 cloves
- Hard cheese 30 g
- Tomato sauceto taste
- Creamy sauceto taste
- Parsleyto taste
- Ground black pepperto taste
- Coarse saltto taste

COOKING INSTRUCTION 15 MINUTES

1. At a loaf (you need a small one, weighing 250-300 grams; a small baguette is suitable), cut off the top part - not with a thin layer, but so that you can then close the sandwich with the cut part. From the bottom, select the crumb. Dry both parts in the oven or in any other acceptable way.

2. Lubricate the lower part inside with tomato sauce: home-made or ketchup - any, to taste. Crush the garlic there.

3. Fill the bottom with a mixture of diced peeled cucumbers and tomatoes, chopped onions, thin straws of ham, grated cheese, green peas and parsley (as well as any other greens to taste). Salt, pepper. Top with cream sauce. Close the top of the rolls.

Cheese, Bacon and Avocado Club Sandwich

INGREDIENTS

- Bacon 4 pieces
- Garlic 1 clove
- Mayonnaise 125 g
- Lemon juice 1 tablespoon
- Tomatoes 2 pieces
- Rustic bread 12 pieces
- Avocado 1 piece
- Swiss cheese 300 g

COOKING INSTRUCTION 30 MINUTES

1. Preheat the grill. Put the bacon and fry for 2 minutes on both sides until golden brown.

2. Meanwhile, mix mayonnaise, chopped garlic, and lemon juice. Add ground black pepper. Put 8 slices of bread on the grill and fry on one side for 1 minute until golden brown.

3. Put 4 toasts on the board, fried side down. Spread with half the garlic mayonnaise, then put the tomatoes sliced in thin circles, then a piece of cheese. On top of the cheese, put a slice of not toasted bread, spreading it with the remaining mayonnaise, then put the bacon.

4. Mash the avocado to a puree condition and lay on top of the mayonnaise. Top with the remaining 4 slices of toasted bread, fried side up. Press the sandwiches lightly. Put 1.5 pieces of cheese on top so that it completely covers the top bread and hangs slightly on the sides.

5. Place the sandwiches under the grill and fry until the cheese is browned. Cool slightly and cut in half diagonally. serve warm.

Turkey club sandwich

INGREDIENTS
- Pancetta 6 pieces
- White bread 6 slices
- Green salad 25 g
- Tomatoes 1 piece
- Chives 2 tablespoons
- Turkey 175 g
- Chopped parsley 1 teaspoon
- Chicken egg 2 pieces
- White wine vinegar 1 tablespoon
- Garlic 1 clove
- Dijon mustard 1 tablespoon
- Olive oil 200 ml
- Saltto taste
- Ground black pepperto taste

COOKING INSTRUCTION 30 MINUTES

1. Preheat the grill. Place the pancetta on the wire rack and fry for 3-4 minutes until crisp. Flip 1 time. Put on a kitchen paper towel and dry.

2. For seasoning, pour in the yolks in a convenient container, add vinegar, mustard, finely chopped garlic, seasonings to taste and mix. Add olive oil while stirring. After a minute, you will notice that the mixture begins to thicken. Start to add oil more actively, stirring constantly, but not too quickly, as the mass may curl.

3. Fry the bread under the grill and spread with the resulting seasoning. Divide the salad between two slices of bread, put the chopped tomatoes and a piece of finely chopped chives. Add seasoning to taste.

4. Put slices of cooked turkey on top, cover with slices of bread with the buttered side up. Put the salad, on top - crispy pancetta and sprinkle with chives. Cover with the remaining slices of bread and gently squeeze. Cut each sandwich into four triangles, pierce with a toothpick so that it does not fall apart. Arrange on serving plates, sprinkle with parsley.

Sandwich with pear, brie and ham

INGREDIENTS
- Whole grain bun 1 piece
- Pears 3 pieces
- Brie cheese 100 g
- Parma ham 3 pieces

COOKING INSTRUCTION 5 MINUTES

1. Cut the bun in half.
2. Lay the **INGREDIENTS** in layers.
3. Lightly heat in a pan.

SNACKS

Hot cheese and onion appetizer

ENERGY VALUE PER PORTION
CALORIE CONTENT 264 KCAL
SQUIRRELS 9,4 GRAM
FATS 23,2 GRAM
CARBOHYDRATES 4.6 GRAM
INGREDIENTS

- Ricotta cheese 120 g
- Mayonnaise 90 g
- Grated Parmesan 60 g
- Sweet onion 1 head
- Freshly ground black pepperto taste

COOKING INSTRUCTION 50 MINUTES

1. Preheat the oven to 180 degrees.
2. In a bowl, mix ricotta, mayonnaise, parmesan, chopped onions and a little
3. Put the onion-cheese mass in a small form and put in the oven for 30-50 minutes until golden brown.

Appetizer of scallops in shells under a cheese crust

ENERGY VALUE PER PORTION
CALORIE CONTENT 428KCAL
SQUIRRELS 26.6 GRAM
FATS 25.3 GRAM
CARBOHYDRATES 19GRAM
INGREDIENTS

- Wheat flour ¼ cup
- ¾ teaspoonsalt
- Curry ½ teaspoon
- Cayenne pepper 0.125 teaspoons
- Scallops 750 g
- Butter6 tablespoons
- Fresh mushrooms 250 g
- Onions 240 g
- Dry white wine 0.6 cups
- Cognac 2 tablespoons
- Crushed crackers 3 tablespoons
- Grated Gruyere cheese 40 g
- Lemon juice 1 tablespoon

COOKING INSTRUCTION 50 MINUTES

1. In a bowl, combine flour, salt, curry and cayenne pepper. Add scallops and mix well.
2. Melt 4 tablespoons of butter in a large skillet over medium heat. Spread the scallops and fry until golden brown for about 4 minutes, turning over 1 time.
3. Pour in the wine and cook for a while, stirring occasionally. Then reduce heat slightly and let the sauce evaporate in half. Remove from heat and pour in cognac.
4. Preheat the grill in the oven.
5. Spread the scallops on the shells from them and put them in a mold.
6. Combine the crackers, the remaining softened butter and the gruyere. Put on top on the scallops. Place under the grill and let brown. Sprinkle with lemon juice and serve immediately.

Mackerel tuna (mackerel) appetizer in marinade

ENERGY VALUE PER PORTION
CALORIE CONTENT 751 KCAL
SQUIRRELS 115.8 GRAM
FATS thirty GRAM
CARBOHYDRATES 4.8 GRAM
INGREDIENTS

- Tuna 1 piece
- Sweet onion 1 piece
- Red bell pepper ½ pieces
- 5 tablespoonsolive oil
- Bay leaf 2 pieces
- ½ teaspoonblack peppercorns
- Saltto taste

COOKING INSTRUCTION 30 MINUTES

1. Put a pot of water on the stove - cook tuna in it. Pour salt, black pepper and bay leaf there.
2. Cut the fish into pieces.
3. Chop finely onion and half a large bell pepper.
4. Cook fish for about 12 minutes. It is very important not to overexpose. Put the prepared pieces on a plate, let them cool. Peel off skin and bones. It's simple - the meat is easily separated from the spine, and there are almost no ribs.
5. Mix the tuna with onions, pepper, salt, pepper and pour over olive oil well. Leave to rest for a couple of hours.

Italian artichoke and black olives appetizer

ENERGY VALUE PER PORTION
CALORIE CONTENT 438 KCAL
SQUIRRELS 5.8 GRAM
FATS 29.8 GRAM
CARBOHYDRATES 34.9 GRAM
INGREDIENTS

- Olive oil 3 tablespoons
- Red onion 2 heads
- Brown soft sugar 1 teaspoon
- Caraway leaves 1 tablespoon
- Balsamic vinegar 1 tablespoon
- Yeast puff pastry 250 g
- Canned Artichokes 170 g
- Pitted olives 16 pieces

COOKING INSTRUCTION 45 MINUTES

1. Heat 2 tablespoons of oil over low heat in a pan. Add onion sliced in half rings and cook, stirring, 15 minutes until soft. Add vinegar and brown sugar and cook for another 15 minutes until light brown. Remove from heat, add chopped caraway seeds and let cool.
2. Preheat the oven to 200 degrees and set the greased baking sheet to heat. Cut 4 mugs of dough with a diameter of 10 cm and lay the onions on them, leaving empty edges of 1.5 cm each.
3. Put the dough on a hot baking sheet and place in the oven for 12-15 minutes until the dough is browned.
4. Top the onion with chopped artichokes and olives. Sprinkle with olive oil on top and garnish with sprigs of caraway seeds.

Greek potato snack with almonds and garlic

ENERGY VALUE PER PORTION
CALORIE CONTENT 488 KCAL
SQUIRRELS 6.7 GRAM
FAT S 39.3 GRAM
CARBOHYDRATES 29 th GRAM
INGREDIENTS

- Potato 340 g
- Almond Flakes 60 g
- Crushed crackers ½ cup
- Garlic 3 cloves
- Water ½ cup
- Lemon juice 4 teaspoons
- Olive oil 0.6 cup
- Crackersto taste

COOKING INSTRUCTION 25 MINUTES

1. Preheat the oven to 180 degrees.
2. Put the peeled potatoes in a pan, fill with water, salt and cook until soft for about 15 minutes.
3. Put the almonds and crackers on a baking sheet and put in the oven for 8-10 minutes until golden brown, sometimes stirring. Chill.
4. In the combine chop the garlic, then add the crackers with almonds and chop again. Then pour water, 1 tablespoon of lemon juice and pour 0.75 teaspoons of salt. Mix well.5. Drain the potatoes and mash with a fork. Transfer in a nut mass to the combine and add olive oil. Grind everything well until smooth and transfer to a bowl. Serve with crackers.

Grilled vegetables appetizer with ricotta

ENERGY VALUE PER PORTION
CALORIE CONTENT 355 KCAL
SQUIRRELS 15,5 GRAM
FATS 21.3 GRAM
CARBOHYDRATES 28.5 GRAM
INGREDIENTS

- Eggplant 2 pieces
- Onion 2 pieces
- Red bell pepper 1 piece
- Green bell pepper 1 piece
- Yellow bell pepper1 piece
- Tomatoes flame 4 pieces
- Champignons 4 pieces
- Ricotta cheese 250 g
- Cilantroto taste
- Olive oil 50 ml
- Soy sauce 2 tablespoons
- Provencal herbsto taste
- Garlic 1 clove
- Lemon ½ pieces
- Tarragon leavesto taste

COOKING INSTRUCTION 40 MINUTES

1. Peel a mixture of fresh herbs from the stems and chop finely with a knife to the state of powder, mix with cottage cheese.
2. Cut the vegetables into slices 1.5–2 cm thick, tomatoes into 2 halves in length, onions into thick rings.

3. Heat the pan well and fry all the vegetables and mushrooms on each side without oil until they turn beautiful.

4. Prepare the marinade by mixing all the INGREDIENTS, and with a brush, saturate them with plenty of vegetables and mushrooms. Put the soaked vegetables in a bowl, cover and let stand for 5-10 minutes. On a dish in a circle, lay out the vegetables, in the center - ricotta mixed with herbs.

Crispy Seed Appetizer

ENERGY VALUE PER PORTION
CALORIE CONTENT 11468 KCAL
SQUIRRELS 457.3 GRAM
FATS 167.2 GRAM
CARBOHYDRATES 2038.8 GRAM
INGREDIENTS

- Sesame seeds ½ cup
- Black sesame seeds ¼ cup
- Poppy seeds 2 tablespoons
- Mustard Seeds 2 Tbsp
- Coarse salt 1 tablespoon
- Cayenne pepper ¾ teaspoon
- Water 6 tablespoons
- Corn starch 2 tablespoons
- Vonton dough 40 pieces
- Vegetable oilto taste

COOKING INSTRUCTION 30 MINUTES

1. In a small bowl, combine sesame seeds, poppy seeds, mustard seeds, salt and cayenne pepper. In another bowl, mix water and starch.

2. In a saucepan, heat the vegetable oil to 180 degrees. Working very quickly, lubricate one side of two slices of dough with starch mixture and roll this side in a mixture with seeds, pressing lightly. Shake off excess and put in oil for 8-10 seconds until golden brown. Lay on a paper towel. Do the same with the

3. Before serving, preheat in an oven preheated to 100 degrees for 10-12 minutes.

Pumpkin appetizer with cranberries and dried apricots

ENERGY VALUE PER PORTION
CALORIE CONTENT 195 KCAL
SQUIRRELS 3.4 GRAM
FATS 12,4 GRAM
CARBOHYDRATES 21.3 GRAM
INGREDIENTS

- Pumpkin squash 500 g
- Extra virgin olive oil 2 tablespoons
- Apple cider vinegar 1 tablespoon
- ¼ teaspoonsalt
- Freshly ground black pepper ¼ teaspoon
- Dried apricots 40 g
- Dried Cranberries 30 g
- Chopped chives 2 tablespoons
- Toasted almond flakes 2 tablespoons

COOKING INSTRUCTION 20 MINUTES

1. Cut the pumpkin lengthwise into 4 pieces, peel the seeds and cut across very thin slices.

2. Steam the pumpkin until soft for 5–7 minutes.

3. In a large bowl, mix vinegar, salt, pepper and olive oil. Add pumpkin, chopped dried apricots and cranberries. Stir, sprinkle with nuts and serve.

Quick appetizers in tartlets

ENERGY VALUE PER PORTION
CALORIE CONTENT 351 KCAL
SQUIRRELS 12 GRAM
FATS 21.7 GRAM
CARBOHYDRATES 26.7 GRAM
INGREDIENTS

- Tartlets 20 pieces
- Zucchini 350 g
- Onions 100 g
- Carrot 100 g
- Tomato paste 1 teaspoon
- Sugar6 teaspoons
- Garlic 3 cloves
- Vegetable oil 50 ml
- Saltto taste
- Water 100 ml
- Apple cider vinegar 50 g
- Soy Sauce 190 ml
- Pork 150 g
- Cucumbers 2 pieces
- Chili pepper 1 g
- Chicken egg 2 pieces
- Cheese 70 g
- Mayonnaise 30 g
- Dillto taste
- Tomatoes 1 piece
- Radish 3 pieces
- Sour cream 2 tablespoons
- Dijon mustardto taste
- Sesame seedsto taste
- Iceberg saladto taste

COOKING INSTRUCTION 1 HOUR

1. Prepare the **INGREDIENTS** for squash caviar. Peel and rinse onions and carrots with cold water.
2. Fry onions and carrots in vegetable oil, turning on a slow fire.
3. Zucchini cut into circles, and then cut into 4 parts.
4. Add the coarsely chopped zucchini and simmer for 30-35 minutes.
5. After a while, add tomato paste and 2 pinches of sugar. Mix thoroughly and simmer for another 10 minutes.
6. Pour in water and cook zucchini caviar until the liquid completely evaporates.
7. Add the grated garlic and salt. Then grind the eggs with a potato masher.
8. For the second snack you will need teriyaki sauce, which we will prepare on our own. Pour apple cider vinegar into the stewpan, add soy sauce and 4 tbsp. tablespoons of sugar. Mix.
9. Let it boil and cook for 30 minutes.
10. Peeled pork fillet cut into small cubes.
11. Transfer the pork into a deep bowl and pour the sauce (1 tbsp. Spoon).
12. Stir and pour the vegetable oil.
13. Turn on the maximum heat and heat the pan. Fry pork in vegetable oil for a maximum of 1 minute. As soon as the juice begins to stand out, remove the meat from the fire. Cool the pork.
14. 2/3 of the cucumber is cut into cubes, and the rest - in thin circles.
15. Hot pepper cut into thin rings.

16. In a bowl we spread pork, cucumber, pepper, a little garlic and pour teriyaki sauce. Mix - and the meat appetizer is ready!

17. We proceed to the preparation of the next filling. Grate the cheese on a coarse grater.

18. Add mayonnaise.

19. There we pour the eggs, grated on a coarse grater, and garlic crushed on a fine grater.

20. Dill finely chopped.

21. Add the greens to the bowl and mix.

22. Now we begin to prepare a vegetable salad. Cut the cucumber into 4 parts, then finely chop.

23. We try to cut radishes as finely as possible.

24. Tomato is also finely chopped.

25. Combine the prepared **INGREDIENTS** in a deep bowl. Add finely chopped dill.

26. We season the summer salad with sour cream.

27. Gradually approach the final stage. We put lettuce leaves on the bottom of five tartlets, place a cucumber on top.

28. On top of the cucumbers spread the meat filling. The next five tartlets are filled with cheese and egg filling.

29. In the penultimate five tartlets put zucchini caviar. The remaining tartlets are filled with vegetable salad, laying lettuce on the bottom. We decorate tartlets with pork with mustard seeds. Sprinkle cheese and egg and squash filling with sesame seeds on top.

Bacon appetizer

ENERGY VALUE PER PORTION
CALORIE CONTENT 343 KCAL
SQUIRRELS 1,5 GRAM
FATS 37.1 GRAM
CARBOHYDRATES 2.2 GRAM
INGREDIENTS

- Salty lard 250 g
- Garlic 5 cloves
- Ground black pepperto taste
- Greensto taste
- Sweet pepper 20 g

COOKING INSTRUCTION 25 MINUTES

1. Lard and garlic through a meat grinder.
2. Finely chop the herbs and pepper.
3. Add ground pepper and mix all the **INGREDIENTS** until smooth.

Zucchini Appetizer with Cashew Sour Cream

ENERGY VALUE PER PORTION
CALORIE CONTENT 514 KCAL
SQUIRRELS 19.9 GRAM
FATS 28,2 GRAM
CARBOHYDRATES 51.7 GRAM
INGREDIENTS

- Cashew 1 cup
- Sea saltto taste
- Zucchini 5 pieces
- Cayenne pepper 1 teaspoon
- Tamarind paste 1 cup

COOKING INSTRUCTION 40 MINUTES + 8 HOURS

1. In a blender, chop nuts with 1 cup of water and salt. Start with 0.5 cups and gradually add even to the consistency of thick sour cream.

2. Cover the mass with gauze and leave for 8 hours or more. During this time, it will acquire the aroma of sour cream and covered with a gray crust. Remove the crust with a spoon, cover the sour cream and put in the refrigerator.

3. Cut the zucchini into small pieces and marinate in cayenne pepper, tamarind paste and a small amount of water for 15 minutes.

4. Put the slices of zucchini on the dryer, put a small amount of sour cream on top of each and dry for 12 hours at 40 degrees until crisp.

Black Bean, Tomato and Avocado Appetizer

ENERGY VALUE PER PORTION
CALORIE CONTENT 387 KCAL
SQUIRRELS 17.6 GRAM
FATS 13.3 GRAM
CARBOHYDRATES 51,2 GRAM
INGREDIENTS

- Black canned beans 900 g
- Roman tomatoes5 pieces
- Onion 1 head
- Avocado 1 piece
- Garlic 3 cloves
- Chopped cilantro (coriander) ¼ cup
- Lime 1 piece
- Corn chipsto taste

COOKING INSTRUCTION 30 MINUTES

1. In a large bowl, mix the dried beans, chopped tomatoes, chopped onion, chopped avocado, chopped garlic, and cilantro.

2. Before serving, squeeze the lime juice on top and serve with corn chips.

Thai appetizer with crabs and avocado

ENERGY VALUE PER PORTION
CALORIE CONTENT 642 KCAL
SQUIRRELS 9.7 GRAM
FATS 56.2 GRAM
CARBOHYDRATES 28 GRAM
INGREDIENTS

- Lime juice 2 tablespoons
- Ginger Root 1 teaspoon
- 5 tablespoonsmayonnaise
- Avocado 1 piece
- White bread 2 slices
- Lemon grass 1 piece
- Crab meat 150 g
- Ground black pepperto taste

COOKING INSTRUCTION 8 MINUTES

1. Combine half of the lime juice with ginger and lemon sorghum. Add mayonnaise and mix. Spread the bread with mayonnaise.

2. Cut the avocado in half, take out the stone and peel it. Cut the pulp into thin slices. Arrange on slices of bread. Sprinkle lime juice on top.

3. Put the finished crab meat on a spoon with a spoon and add the remaining lime juice. Add the remaining mayonnaise and sprinkle with black pepper. Garnish with fresh coriander and serve.

Halibut appetizer with carrots, fennel, lemon and garlic

ENERGY VALUE PER PORTION
CALORIE CONTENT 464 KCAL
SQUIRRELS 39.5 GRAM
FATS 31.6 GRAM
CARBOHYDRATES 6.5 GRAM
INGREDIENTS

- Olive oil 1 cup
- Fennel root 1 piece
- Lemon 2 pieces
- Halibut fillet 8 pieces
- 2 carrots
- Cherry Tomatoes 340 g
- Fresh thyme 2 bunches
- Garlic 2 cloves

COOKING INSTRUCTION 30 MINUTES + 5 MINUTES

1. Preheat the oven to 230 degrees. Cover the large baking sheet with foil, leaving long edges. Lubricate the foil with 1 spoon of oil.
2. Put thinly sliced fennel on the foil evenly. Then layer thinly sliced lemons and top the fish. Salt and pepper.
3. Sprinkle the carrots with chopped straws on top and lay out the cherry cut in half.
4. Then lay out 16 branches of thyme, wrap in foil and put in the oven until cooked, for about 12 minutes.
5. Meanwhile, in a blender, whisk the remaining olive oil with chopped garlic. Salt and pepper.
6. Carefully open the foil and sprinkle the fish and vegetables with oil sauce. Wrap the foil and let the fish cool for 1 hour. Then put in the refrigerator overnight.
7. Remove the thyme sprigs. Transfer 1 piece of fish to each plate along with vegetables and sauce. Garnish with lemon slices.

Persimmon and Parma ham appetizer

ENERGY VALUE PER PORTION
CALORIE CONTENT 136 KCAL
SQUIRRELS 7. 3GRAM
FATS 5.8 GRAM
CARBOHYDRATES 16.9 GRAM
INGREDIENTS

- Persimmon 2 pieces
- Fresh mint 1 bunch
- Arugula 1 bunch
- Honey 1 tablespoon
- Balsamic sauce 1 teaspoon
- Parma ham 100 g

COOKING INSTRUCTION 15 MINUTES

1. Persimmon cut into slices.
2. Finely chop the mint and arugula, add a tablespoon of honey and a teaspoon of balsamic sauce.
3. Put greens on slices of persimmons, wrap all Parma ham.

Eggplant, cucumber and sweet pepper appetizer

ENERGY VALUE PER PORTION
CALORIE CONTENT 330 KCAL
SQUIRRELS 18,4 GRAM
FATS 17.3 GRAM
CARBOHYDRATES 26.3 GRAM

INGREDIENTS

- Eggplant 2 pieces
- Vegetable oilto taste
- Cream cheese 2 pieces
- Chicken egg 2 pieces
- Garlic 4 cloves
- Mayonnaise 2 tablespoons
- Sweet pepper ¼ pieces
- Cucumbers 1 piece
- 12 pitted olives
- Saltto taste
- Ground black pepperto taste

COOKING INSTRUCTION 1 HOUR

1. Hard boiled eggs.

2. We cut eggplants in circles up to 1 cm thick.

3. Fry eggplant in preheated vegetable oil on both sides, over moderate heat, until light brown.

4. Immediately spread on a napkin to absorb excess oil. Let the eggplant cool. We don't salt the eggplants, since then on top we will have a rather spicy salad.

5. For the salad, grate on a fine grater processed cheese (they should be kept in the refrigerator to better rub) and boiled eggs. We sell garlic through the press. Salt and pepper to taste, mix and season with mayonnaise. Salad mass should be quite thick.

Chicken Breast Appetizer

INGREDIENTS

- Chicken breast 1 piece
- Soy sauce 2 tablespoons
- Garli c4 cloves
- Bay leaf 4 pieces
- Suneli hops 2 teaspoons
- Saltto taste
- Freshly ground black pepperto taste

COOKING INSTRUCTION 3 HOURS 25 MINUTES

1. Wash, dry the chicken breast, peel it (do not throw it out), and cut it to form aroll: you should get two large pieces 1 cm thick (if the pieces are not completely even or more than two pieces are obtained, it's okay, the main thing is to make it was possible to form a roll).

2. Salt the chicken, pepper and lightly beat.

4. Rub the garlic on a fine grater or squeeze through a press, finely break the bay leaf.

5. After the chicken is marinated, spread it on the board, sprinkle with suneli hops, bay leaf, grated garlic.

6. Form a roll, wrap the breast on top of the skin. It's impossible to completely wrap the roll with skin.

7. Then wrap the roll in foil and send in an oven preheated to 200 degrees for 40 minutes. Place the roll on a baking sheet so that the side with the skin is on top.

8. After 40 minutes, cut the foil on top and open the roll, continue to bake for another 15 minutes so that it is browned.

9. Use roll should be chilled.

Dried beef and cheese appetizer

ENERGY VALUE PER PORTION
CALORIE CONTENT 283 KCAL
SQUIRRELS 21.7 GRAM
FATS 21 GRAM
CARBOHYDRATES 2,4 GRAM

INGREDIENTS

- Mayonnaise 3 tablespoons
- Sour cream 3 tablespoons
- Saltto taste
- Beef jerky 150 g
- Ground black pepperto taste
- Onion 40 g
- Grated cheese 100 g

COOKING INSTRUCTION 10 MINUTES

1. Pass the beef through a meat grinder or blender along with onions, add mayonnaise, sour cream and grated cheese. Stir, salt, pepper and refrigerate before eating.
2. Serve with bread rolls, crackers or toast.

Salmon appetizer with tartar sauce and pink pepper

ENERGY VALUE PER PORTION
CALORIE CONTENT 385 KCAL
SQUIRRELS 40.7 GRAM
FATS 22.2 GRAM
CARBOHYDRATES 2,4 GRAM
INGREDIENTS

- Mayonnaise 100 g
- Sour cream 65 g
- Red onion 60 g
- Chopped parsley 20 g
- Capers 300 g
- Pink pepper 2 teaspoons
- Salmon fillet 1.6 kg

COOKING INSTRUCTION 30 MINUTES + 5 MINUTES

1. In a small bowl, mix mayonnaise, sour cream, finely chopped red onion, parsley, capers, and chopped pink pepper. Salt and pepper. Cover with wrap and refrigerate for 1 day.
2. Preheat the grill and lightly grease with vegetable oil. Cut the fish into thin slices, salt and pepper and fry in portions for 2 minutes without turning the fish over. Put on a dish, cover with foil and send in the refrigerator for the night.
3. Put the fish in a dish, leave for 1 hour before serving and serve with tartar sauce.

Chicken appetizer with garlic, mayonnaise and walnuts

ENERGY VALUE PER PORTION
CALORIE CONTENT 483 KCAL
SQUIRRELS 35 GRAM
FATS 37,4 GRAM
CARBOHYDRATES3.4GRAM
INGREDIENTS

- Chicken breast fillet 300 g
- Cheese 200 g
- Greens 1 bunch
- Walnuts 130 g
- Garlicto taste
- Mayonnaiseto taste
- Olivesto taste

COOKING INSTRUCTION 40 MINUTES

1. Boil the chicken breast fillet in salted water (15-20 minutes) and finely chop.
2. Three cheese on a fine grater. Finely chop the greens. We chop walnuts. Add crushed garlic. Just mix all the **INGREDIENTS** and season with mayonnaise.

3. Roll the balls from the resulting mass. Bone in nut crumbs, make "fastenings" from halves of olives, and loops from greens.

Blackcurrant herring appetizer

ENERGY VALUE PER PORTION
CALORIE CONTENT 357 KCAL
SQUIRRELS 14.6 GRAM
FATS 27,2 GRAM
CARBOHYDRATES 12.8 GRAM
INGREDIENTS

- Norwegian slightly salted herring 1 piece
- Cream 35%200 ml
- ½ bunchgreen onions
- Sugar 1 teaspoon
- Red onion 1 head
- Blackcurrant 200 g
- Lemon juice 1 teaspoon
- Ground black pepperto taste

COOKING INSTRUCTION 30 MINUTES
1. Peel herring from skin and viscera, disassemble on fillet and remove bones. Cut the fillet into small pieces.
2. Finely chop the green and red onions. Add sugar, lemon juice, black pepper and pour cream.
3. All move well, add pieces of herring and currants. Mix well again and pepper to taste.
4. Refrigerate for several hours (or overnight).
5. Put the prepared appetizer in a bowl or cup, garnish with currant berries and a piece of herring.

Vegetable appetizer with ham and eggs Amanita

ENERGY VALUE PER PORTION
CALORIE CONTENT 128 KCAL
SQUIRRELS 7 GRAM
FATS 10.3 GRAM
CARBOHYDRATES 1.9 GRAM
INGREDIENTS

- Ham 120 g
- Cheese 100 g
- Cherry Tomatoes 15 pieces
- Mayonnaise 2 tablespoons
- Greens 1 bunch
- Chicken egg 3 pieces
- Cucumbers 2 pieces

COOKING INSTRUCTION 25 MINUTES
1. We rub boiled eggs and cheese on a fine grater. Cut the ham into small cubes. In a deep cup, mix the eggs, cheese, ham and mayonnaise. Cherry tomatoes are cut in half. Cucumber cut into rings half a centimeter thick. All the components of the snack are ready, it remains to assemble them into the original composition.
2. On a flat dish we spread chopped greens, which will serve as a clearing for fly agaric. Greens will suit absolutely any that is at your fingertips: onions, dill, parsley, etc. On top of the greens we spread the pieces of cucumbers, which will be the basis for the mushrooms. From a mixture of eggs, cheese and ham, we form small balls. If you add such a ball to the top and bottom, you get a barrel that will serve as the leg of the mushroom. We sit the resulting legs on the cucumbers. From above we put on red hats made of halves of cherry tomatoes. To give the already beautiful appetizer a finished look, it remains only to draw white dots from mayonnaise on red hats. This is most conveniently done with a regular toothpick.

Three types of cheese snacks with crackers

ENERGY VALUE PER PORTION
CALORIE CONTENT 673 KCAL
SQUIRRELS 21,4 GRAM
FATS 49.8 GRAM
CARBOHYDRATES 42.8 GRAM
INGREDIENTS

- Butter 120 g
- Cream Cheese 600 g
- Lemon juice 2 tablespoons
- Worcestershire sauce ½ teaspoon
- Ground red pepper ¼ teaspoon
- Sea saltto taste
- Ground white pepper ½ teaspoon
- Dried Cranberries 150 g
- Cheddar Cheese 300 g
- Ginger Apple Chutney 40 g
- Shallots 1 head
- Feta cheese 200 g
- Ground Pecan 170 g
- Goat cheese 200 g
- Chives 35 g
- Parsley 25 g
- Crackers 500 g

COOKING INSTRUCTION 1 HOUR 15 MINUTES

1. Mix the butter (room temperature), cream cheese, lemon juice, Worcestershire sauce, red pepper, salt and white pepper in a large bowl until smooth.
2. Divide the mixture evenly into three separate bowls.
3. In the first bowl add grated cheddar cheese, cranberries and chutney (see the recipe on my page) and mix well.
4. In the second bowl add chopped feta, shallots and chopped pecans - mix well.
5. In a third bowl add goat cheese, chopped green onions and chopped parsley - mix well.
6. Spread cling film on the desktop, put 1 type of snack on it, roll it up and give it the desired shape with your hands. Repeat the same with the 2 remaining snacks. Put in the refrigerator for 1 hour.
7. Prepare a dish large enough to serve three types of cheese and crackers.
8. Carefully unfold the snacks and place them on the dish along with crackers (different types can be).
9. Before serving, decorate using all your creativity!

Vegetable snack

ENERGY VALUE PER PORTION
CALORIE CONTENT 259 KCAL
SQUIRRELS 2.6 GRAM
FATS 25,2 GRAM
CARBOHYDRATES 7.7 GRAM
INGREDIENTS

- Zucchini 1 piece
- Avocado 1 piece
- Olive oil 50 ml
- Cucumbers 1 piece
- Sea saltto taste
- Paprika ¼ teaspoon

- Dried tarragonpinch

COOKING INSTRUCTION 15 MINUTES

1. Cut the zucchini, cucumber and avocado into pieces.
2. Mix all the **INGREDIENTS**

Smoked turkey appetizer with cheese sauce and croutons

INGREDIENTS

- Smoked Turkey 200 g
- Parmesan Cheese 100 g
- Philadelphia cheese 20 g
- Mascarpone cheese 4 tablespoons
- Greens 1 bunch
- Olive paste 2 teaspoons
- Lemon 1 piece
- Cream 2 tablespoons
- 2 piecebread toast
- Saltto taste
- Ground black pepperto taste

COOKING INSTRUCTION 15 MINUTES

1. Cook the cheese sauce. To do this, mix grated parmesan with Philadelphia, mascarpone, salt, pepper, herbs and cream.
2. Toast the toasts. Drizzle with oil.
3. Cut the smoked turkey fillet into thin slices and place on plates. Top with olive paste and drizzle with lemon. Sprinkle with green onions.
4. Serve with sauce and toast.

Hot appetizer of spinach and artichokes with cheese

ENERGY VALUE PER PORTION
CALORIE CONTENT 287 KCAL
SQUIRRELS 12.9 GRAM
FATS 22.5 GRAM
CARBOHYDRATES 14.5 GRAM
INGREDIENTS

- Frozen Spinach 300 g
- Canned artichoke cores 400 g
- Ricotta cheese 120 g
- Sour cream 5 tablespoons
- Garlic1 clove
- Mayonnaise 45 g
- ½ teaspoonchili sauce
- Grated Parmesan Cheese 30 g
- Mozzarella Cheese 60 g

COOKING INSTRUCTION 50 MINUTES

1. Preheat the oven to 180 degrees.
2. Defrost spinach and chop finely. Transfer to a bowl.
3. Add finely chopped artichokes, ricotta, sour cream, mayonnaise, chopped garlic, chili sauce, parmesan and grated mozzarella. Put everything in a small form and bake for 20-40 minutes until golden brown.

Zucchini and tomato appetizer with cheese

ENERGY VALUE PER PORTION
CALORIE CONTENT 170 KCAL
SQUIRRELS 9.6 GRAM
FATS 10 GRAM
CARBOHYDRATES 10.8 GRAM
INGREDIENTS

- Carrot 1 piece
- Cheese 130 g
- Garlic 4 cloves
- Mayonnaiseto taste
- Zucchini 1 piece
- Tomatoes 3 pieces

COOKING INSTRUCTION 25 MINUTES

1. Zucchini or zucchini cut into rings about 1 cm thick, roll in flour, fry on both sides in vegetable oil.
2. Tomatoes cut into rings about 0.5 cm thick.
3. Grate carrots and cheese. Mix, add garlic (via press), mayonnaise.
4. Put zucchini on a dish, put tomato rings on top (add a little salt), and cheese and carrot mixture on top.

Caramelized onion, ricotta and parmesan hot appetizer

ENERGY VALUE PER PORTION
CALORIE CONTENT 386 KCAL
SQUIRRELS 10.7 GRAM
FATS 32.6 GRAM
CARBOHYDRATES 14 GRAM
INGREDIENTS

- Butter 1 tablespoon
- Sweet bow 4 heads
- Vegetable oil 1 tablespoon
- Ricotta cheese 120 g
- Mayonnaise 90 g
- Grated Parmesan 60 g
- Freshly ground white pepperto taste

COOKING INSTRUCTION 30 MINUTES

1. Remove from heat and transfer to a bowl. Add ricotta, mayonnaise, parmesan and pepper. Mix everything well and put in a refractory form.
2. Bake 30-50 minutes until golden brown.
3. Melt the butter in a pan and add the vegetable oil. Add the onion thinly sliced in half rings and cook over low heat until the onion begins to caramelize, about 1-2 hours.
4. Preheat the oven to 180 degrees.

Appetizer stuffed with goat cheese piquillo
ENERGY VALUE PER PORTION
CALORIE CONTENT 416 KCAL
SQUIRRELS 12 GRAM
FATS 38.3 GRAM
CARBOHYDRATES 6 GRAM
INGREDIENTS

- Soft goat cheese 100 g
- Peeled Pikyo Peppers 150 g
- Garlic 1 clove
- Mustard oil 3 tablespoons

- Sea saltto taste
- Ground black pepperto taste

COOKING INSTRUCTION 15 MINUTES

1. Preheat the oven to 200 degrees.
2. Carefully pour peeled peppers with goat cheese using a teaspoon so that the filling does not fall out. Grind the garlic with a knife or using a garlic press. Put peppers on a baking sheet, sprinkle with salt, pepper, garlic and pour mustard oil so that the surface of each pepper is well covered with oil.
3. Place the pan in a well preheated oven for 7-10 minutes.

Omelet appetizer with herring and cream cheese

ENERGY VALUE PER PORTION
CALORIE CONTENT 532 KCAL
SQUIRRELS 23.6 GRAM
FATS 39.9 GRAM
CARBOHYDRATES 20.5 GRAM
INGREDIENTS

- Potato 4 pieces
- Herring 300 g
- Cream cheese 4 tablespoons
- Dill 1 bunch
- Garlic 1 clove
- Vegetable oil 2 tablespoons
- Ground black pepperpinch
- ½ teaspoonsea salt

COOKING INSTRUCTION 30 MINUTES

1. Peel potatoes, cut into slices and fry in vegetable oil.
2. Beat eggs with a pinch of salt.
3. Peel and grind the garlic with a pinch of salt and pepper into the pulp with the flat side of the knife.
4. Fry the potatoes with a fork, add the garlic and beaten eggs, mix everything.
5. Heat the remaining vegetable oil in a pan, put the potato and egg mass, cover and fry for 3 minutes. Turn over and fry the omelet on the other side for another 2-3 minutes.

Fried Tomato and Herb Appetizer

ENERGY VALUE PER PORTION
CALORIE CONTENT 728 KCAL
SQUIRRELS 22.5 GRAM
FATS 10 GRAM
CARBOHYDRATES 134.5 GRAM
INGREDIENTS

- Cherry Tomatoes 1 kg
- Shallots 4 heads
- Red pepper flakes ¼ teaspoon
- Balsamic vinegar 2 teaspoons
- Marjoram 2 tablespoons
- Ciabatta 1 kg
- Olive oilto taste

COOKING INSTRUCTION 1 HOUR

1. Preheat the oven to 190 degrees.
2. In a bowl, mix the half-sliced tomatoes, 0.25 cups of olive oil, very finely chopped shallots, vinegar and red pepper. Transfer to a glass refractory mold. put in the oven for about 45 minutes, until the tomatoes are soft and give juice, sometimes mix. Add marjoram, salt and pepper.
3. Cut the ciabatta horizontally in half, lightly sprinkle with olive oil and put the cut sides up on a baking sheet. Put the tomato mixture on top and put in the oven for about 10 minutes, until the bread becomes

crispy. Put on a board, sprinkle with a small amount of marjoram and black pepper. Cut into small pieces.

Mushroom cold appetizer with lemons

ENERGY VALUE PER PORTION
CALORIE CONTENT7 0 KCAL
SQUIRRELS 6.6 GRAM
FATS 2.7 GRAM
CARBOHYDRATES 5.3 GRAM
INGREDIENTS

- Ceps 150 g
- Lemon 1 piece
- Saltpinch
- Ground black pepperpinch

COOKING INSTRUCTION 20 MINUTES
1. Heat the butter in a pan.
2. Wash and chop the mushrooms into large slices.
3. For 7-10 minutes, fry the mushrooms over medium heat, adding salt and pepper.
4. Cut the lemon into slices, add to the mushrooms, mix, reduce heat to a minimum, cover and leave for 10-15 minutes.
5. Separate the mushrooms from the lemons, transfer the mushrooms to a bowl, cool, put in the refrigerator for 1-2 hours. Serve cold.

Pear, cabbage and tuna appetizer

ENERGY VALUE PER PORTION
CALORIE CONTENT 208 KCAL
SQUIRRELS 8 GRAM
FATS 9 GRAM
CARBOHYDRATES 27.1 GRAM
INGREDIENTS

- Islands Sauce 120 g
- Canned tuna in its own juice 100 g
- Pumpkin seeds 4 teaspoons
- Onions ½ heads
- Red cabbage 80 g
- Pears 4 pieces

COOKING INSTRUCTION 15 MINUTES
1. Wash the pear, cut off the top.
2. Remove the pulp with an ice cream spoon.
3. Cut the pulp of the pear into small cubes.
4. Chop the cabbage.
5. Chop the onion finely.
6. Combine cabbage, pear and tuna.
7. Knead the fish with a fork.
8. Add onion.
9. Fry pumpkin seeds in a dry pan for 1-2 minutes.
10. Pour to the filling, mix.
11. Season with sauce.
12. Stuff the pear.

Christmas salmon and ginger appetizer

ENERGY VALUE PER PORTION
CALORIE CONTENT 278 KCAL
SQUIRRELS 27.7 GRAM

FATS 13.3 GRAM
CARBOHYDRATES 10.3 GRAM
INGREDIENTS

- Salmon Fillet 500 g
- Green onion feathers 2 pieces
- Ginger Root 1 piece
- Lime 1 piece
- Soy sauce 2 tablespoons
- Chives 1 bunch
- Fish sauce 1 tablespoon
- Sesame oil 1 tablespoon

COOKING INSTRUCTION 20 MINUTES
1. Cut the fish into small cubes.
2. Rinse the lime well and grate the zest on a fine grater. Squeeze the juice out of half the lime.
3. Peel a small piece of ginger and chop finely.
4. Finely chop the green onions and chives.
5. In a large bowl, mix ginger with juice and lime zest, chopped green onions and chives, soy and fish sauces and sesame oil.
6. Add fish and mix well.
7. Leave for 10 minutes to marinate in the refrigerator and try to eat for 30 minutes.

Appetizer of green peas, mushrooms and canned peppers

ENERGY VALUE PER PORTION
CALORIE CONTENT 213 KCAL
SQUIRRELS 10.6 GRAM
FATS 10.6 GRAM
CARBOHYDRATES 27.5 GRAM
INGREDIENTS

- Butter 2 tablespoons
- Celery stalk 1 piece
- Onion 60 g
- Frozen Green Peas 2 cups
- Canned Mushrooms 70 g
- Canned Capsicum 60 g

COOKING INSTRUCTION 10 MINUTES \
1. Melt the butter in a skillet over medium heat.
2. Add finely chopped celery and finely chopped onions and sauté until almost tender.
3. Add finely chopped mushrooms, green peas (thawed), and chopped peppers. Fry for a few minutes until all **INGREDIENTS** are well warmed up.

Herring appetizer

ENERGY VALUE PER PORTION
CALORIE CONTENT 198 KCAL
SQUIRRELS 16.7 GRAM
FATS 12.6 GRAM
CARBOHYDRATES 4.8 GRAM
INGREDIENTS

- Lightly salted herring 400 g
- Red onions ½ heads
- Dillto taste
- Sunflower oilto taste

COOKING INSTRUCTION 30 MINUTES
1. Cut herring into small pieces.

2. Onion cut into thin half rings.
3. Chop the dill.
4. Mix all the **INGREDIENTS** and season with oil.

Summer light snack of chicken, greens and mozzarella

ENERGY VALUE PER PORTION
CALORIE CONTENT 711 KCAL
SQUIRRELS 66.9 GRAM
FATS 50.7 GRAM
CARBOHYDRATES 5.3 GRAM
INGREDIENTS

- red cherry tomatoes
- Salad mix "Food" 1 piece
- Roasted cashew nuts1 tablespoon
- Mozzarella Cheese 200 g
- Chicken fille t2 pieces
- 2 tablespoonsolive oil
- Ground black pepperto taste
- Saltto taste
- Soy sauceto taste

COOKING INSTRUCTION 20 MINUTES
1. Cut the chicken into small pieces. Dip them in a mixture of olive oil, pepper, salt and soy sauce. Put the slices in a preheated pan by adding a tablespoon of olive oil. Fry until golden brown.
2. Put salad mixture on the dish, salt, pepper, pour soy sauce to taste, add a tablespoon of olive oil. Top with tomatoes, mozzarella, cut into large pieces. Sprinkle with chopped nuts.
3. Put everything together on a dish and serve until the chicken has cooled.

Beetroot and herring strawberries (Estonian appetizer)

ENERGY VALUE PER PORTION
CALORIE CONTENT 557 KCAL
SQUIRRELS 27.8 GRAM
FATS 40.3 GRAM
CARBOHYDRATES 23.5 GRAM
INGREDIENTS

- Potato 4 pieces
- Beets1 piece
- Herring 2 pieces
- Parsley 1 bunch
- Saltto taste
- Ground black pepperto taste
- Sesame seedsto taste

COOKING INSTRUCTION 30 MINUTES + 40 MINUTES
1. Boil medium-sized potatoes, crush with a fork.
2. Boil a small beet and grate.
3. Salted herring finely, finely chopped.
4. Stir potatoes and beets with each other until a uniform color, salt, pepper to taste.
5. Take a mass with the size of a dessert or tablespoon, make a deepening and put a little herring and form an oval shape similar to strawberries.
6. From the leaves of parsley make a strawberry tail and stick from the wider side, lightly sprinkle with sesame seeds.
7. Strawberry is ready.

Sweet onion and cilantro appetizer

ENERGY VALUE PER PORTION
CALORIE CONTENT 17 KCAL
SQUIRRELS 0.7 GRAM
FATS 0 GRAM
CARBOHYDRATES 4.1 GRAM
INGREDIENTS

- Cilantro (coriander) leaves ¼ cup
- Sweet onion 1 piece
- Chives 1 bunch
- Lime ½ pieces

COOKING INSTRUCTION 10 MINUTES

1. In a small bowl, mix finely chopped sweet onions, finely chopped green onions, cilantro, and half lime juice.

Puff mushroom appetizer with cheeses and green onions

ENERGY VALUE PER PORTION
CALORIE CONTENT 534 KCAL
SQUIRRELS 37.5 GRAM
FATS 35 GRAM
CARBOHYDRATES 20.8 GRAM
INGREDIENTS

- Fresh mushrooms3 cups
- ½ cupcrackers
- Butter 2 tablespoons
- Green onion feathers 75 g
- Monterey Cheese Jack 50 g
- Cottage cheese 2 cups
- ½ cupcheddar cheese
- Chicken egg 2 pieces
- Paprika ¼ teaspoon
- Cayenne pepper ¼ teaspoon

COOKING INSTRUCTION 25 MINUTES

1. Preheat the oven to 180 degrees.

2. In a pan, melt 1 tablespoon of butter and fry the finely chopped mushrooms until soft.

3. Meanwhile, put the crackers in a bag and chop (or chop in a blender) and add to the mushrooms. Stir well and remove from heat.

4. Put the mushroom mixture on the bottom of a round shape.

5. Melt another spoonful of butter in a pan and fry the finely chopped onions until soft. Put on mushrooms in an even layer.

6. Top with grated cheeses.

7. In a blender, mix cottage cheese, eggs and cayenne pepper until smooth. Put on top on the cheese and smooth.

8. Sprinkle paprika on top.

9. Bake for 25-30 minutes. Cool for 10-15 minutes and cut into pieces.

Potato appetizer with mussels

ENERGY VALUE PER PORTION
CALORIE CONTENT 379 KCAL
SQUIRRELS 14.9 GRAM
FATS 25.1 GRAM
CARBOHYDRATES 22 GRAM

INGREDIENTS

- Potato 4 pieces
- Shrimp 50 g
- Mussels 150 g
- Cream 30%150 ml
- Dry white wine 50 ml
- Hard cheese 100 g
- Garlic 2 cloves
- Dill ½ beam
- Saltto taste
- Ground paprikapinch
- 1 tablespoonolive oil

COOKING INSTRUCTION 1 HOUR

1. Boil potatoes in salt water, pour over cold water and peel.
2. Cut across. Cut off the "buttocks" a little to give the cups stability. Then carefully remove the middle with a spoon.
3. Heat olive oil in a frying pan, brown 2 cloves of garlic (pre-crush the garlic).
Remove the garlic and add the prepared mussels and shrimps.
Aluminum frying pan
4. Salt and cook for 1-2 minutes, add dill and remove from heat.
5. Prepare the sauce. Add cream, wine, grated cheese, salt (if necessary).
6. Add sauce to seafood and mix.
7. Grease the cups with olive oil inside and out, salt and stuff with seafood.
8. Place the glasses on a baking sheet and send into the oven at a temperature of 180 degrees. 10-15 minutes, until the cheese is lightly browned on top.
9. Serve hot, garnished with lemon, herbs and sprinkled with paprika.

Baked pumpkin appetizer with red onion and rosemary

INGREDIENTS

- Pumpkin squash 1 kg
- Extra virgin olive oil 2 tablespoons
- Red onion 1 head
- Saltto taste
- Fresh chopped rosemary 1 teaspoon
- Maple Syrup 1 tablespoon
- Dijon mustard 1 tablespoon

COOKING INSTRUCTION 45 MINUTES

1. Preheat the oven to 220 degrees.
2. Peel and finely chop the onion. Cut the pumpkin lengthwise into 4 parts, peel the seeds and cut very thinly across. Put everything in a bowl and add 1 tablespoon of olive oil and salt. Shuffle. Put in 1 layer on a baking sheet.
3. Put in the oven for about 30 minutes until soft and golden.

4. Meanwhile, in a bowl, mix the remaining oil, rosemary. maple syrup and mustard. Add the pumpkin and mix.

Turkey appetizer with fish sauce

ENERGY VALUE PER PORTION
CALORIE CONTENT 481 KCAL
SQUIRRELS 68.5 GRAM
FATS18.5 GRAM
CARBOHYDRATES6.4 GRAM

INGREDIENTS

- Turkey 800 g
- Carrot 1 piece
- Onion 1 head
- Celery 1 piece
- Bay leaf 1 piece
- Canned tuna in oil 400 g
- Capers 20 g
- Dry white wine 100 ml
- Anchovies 4 pieces
- Wine Vinegar 20 ml
- Mayonnaise 5 teaspoons
- Saltto taste
- Ground black pepperto taste

COOKING INSTRUCTION 40 MINUTES

1. Cut carrots and celery and bring to a boil in a large amount of water with salt, vinegar and bay leaf. Boil turkey in this broth.
2. Cut the turkey fillet into very thin slices and serve with the sauce.
3. To prepare the sauce, grind tuna with anchovies and capers in a blender. Mix the resulting mass with wine and mayonnaise.

Appetizer of canned fish and eggs

ENERGY VALUE PER PORTION
CALORIE CONTENT 143 KCAL
SQUIRRELS 17 GRAM
FATS 6.8 GRAM
CARBOHYDRATES 3.3 GRAM
INGREDIENTS

- Chicken egg 2 pieces
- Onion 1 head
- Mayonnaiseto taste
- Pink salmon canned in own juice1 can

COOKING INSTRUCTION 10 MINUTES

1. Hard-boiled eggs. To clear. Cut into small cubes.
2. Canned fish free from bones.
3. Dice the onion. Scald with boiling water to get rid of the pungent odor.
4. Mix everything, add mayonnaise (I add quite a bit), mix everything thoroughly.

Bruschetta with tomatoes

ENERGY VALUE PER PORTION
CALORIE CONTENT 132 KCAL
SQUIRRELS 2,3 GRAM
FATS 7.8 GRAM
CARBOHYDRATES13.1GRAM
INGREDIENTS

- White bread 4 slices
- Tomatoes 3 pieces
- Olive oil 30 ml
- Garlic 3 cloves
- Balsamic cream 10 g
- Freshly ground black pepperto taste
- Saltto taste

- Greens 30 g

COOKING INSTRUCTION 10 MINUTES

1. Fry the bread in a dry frying pan or in the oven until golden brown. In the oven, it will take three to five minutes (depending on the size of a loaf of bread) at a temperature of 200 degrees.

2. Tomatoes cut into cubes with an edge about half a centimeter. Finely chop three cloves of garlic.

3. Heat the pan, pour a little olive oil into it and pour tomatoes and garlic into it. Cook them for a minute or two, just to warm them up without losing the taste of fresh tomato. Then drip into a pan of balsamic cream, mix and remove from heat.

4. Soak the toasted bread with the remaining olive oil, spilling a little on each slice. Put warm tomatoes on top, salt to taste, sprinkle with freshly ground black pepper and finely chopped greens - any that is at hand. And serve as a snack - for example, to wine.

Green Pea Appetizer with Oregano

ENERGY VALUE PER PORTION
CALORIE CONTENT 118 KCAL
SQUIRRELS 8.2 GRAM
FATS 3.2 GRAM
CARBOHYDRATES 20.8 GRAM
INGREDIENTS

- Green peas 500 g
- Coarse saltto taste
- ½ tablespoonbutter
- Fresh chopped oregano leaves1 tablespoon

COOKING INSTRUCTION 30 MINUTES

1. Put peas in a pan and pour a glass of water. Salt and bring to a boil. Cook for 3-4 minutes until the water evaporates.

2. Add the butter and cook for about 2 minutes, until the peas are soft, but remain slightly crispy inside.

3. Remove from heat and mix in oregano. Put on a dish and serve.

Eggplant Puff Appetizer

ENERGY VALUE PER PORTION
CALORIE CONTENT 604 KCAL
SQUIRRELS 7.6 GRAM
FATS 57.9 GRAM
CARBOHYDRATES 13, 2GRAM
INGREDIENTS

- Eggplant 3 pieces
- Tomatoes 3 pieces
- Chicken egg 2 pieces
- Greens 1 bunch
- Chopped garlic 3 cloves
- Mayonnaise 100 g
- Saltto taste
- Vegetable oil 150 ml
- Ground black pepperto taste

COOKING INSTRUCTION 15 MINUTES

1. Cut eggplant into circles, dip in an egg with salt and fry in a pan in oil on both sides, let the oil drain.

2. Cut the tomatoes into slices, chop the herbs and garlic finely and mix with mayonnaise.

3. Lay out on a plate in layers alternately, lubricating each layer with a mixture of mayonnaise.

Appetizer with cottage cheese and smoked fish

INGREDIENTS

- Soft curd 80 g
- Hot smoked mackere l50 g

- Greensto taste
- Green onionsto taste
- Saltto taste
- Sour cream 2 tablespoons
- Borodino bread 1 piece

COOKING INSTRUCTION 20 MINUTES

1. Remove all bones from the fish.
2. Mix cottage cheese, fish, salt, sour cream in a blender until smooth.
3. Then transfer the mixture to a convenient dish, add chopped herbs and green onions, mix everything with a spoon.
4. A snack is pre-spread with a slice of bread.

Mozzarella, tomato and basil appetizer

ENERGY VALUE PER PORTION
CALORIE CONTENT 393 KCAL
SQUIRRELS 18.3 GRAM
FATS 31.1 GRAM
CARBOHYDRATES 8.6 GRAM
INGREDIENTS

- Tomatoes 3 pieces
- Bocconcini Cheese 250 g
- Basil leaves 16 pieces
- Olive oil 3 tablespoons

COOKING INSTRUCTION 20 MINUTES

1. Cut the tomatoes into 1 cm thick circles to make 12 slices. Cut the boccini into 24 pieces 1 cm thick.
2. Put the tomatoes on serving plates, put 2 slices of cheese on top. Put a basil leaf between 2 slices of cheese.
3. Top with oil, sprinkle with chopped basil and salt.

Appetizer lecho

ENERGY VALUE PER PORTION
CALORIE CONTENT 425 KCAL
SQUIRRELS 4.3 GRAM
FATS 23.5 GRAM
CARBOHYDRATES 48.8 GRAM
INGREDIENTS

- Tomatoes 1 kg
- Sweet pepper 1 kg
- Sugar ½ cup
- Salt1 tablespoon
- Acetic acid2 teaspoons
- Vegetable oil ½ cup
- Garlicto taste

COOKING INSTRUCTION 30 MINUTES

1. Wash tomatoes, rinse with boiling water, remove the skin. Cut into strips with peeled peppers.
2. Chop the garlic. Add the rest of the **INGREDIENTS**.
3. Stew for 25–35 minutes until the vegetables are tender (try ready).
4. Roll up in sterile jars.

Ajapsandali snack

ENERGY VALUE PER PORTION
CALORIE CONTENT 69 KCAL
SQUIRRELS 2.6 GRAM
FATS 0.3 GRAM

CARBOHYDRATES 14.9 GRAM
INGREDIENTS
- Tomatoes 1 kg
- Onion 5 heads
- Sea saltto taste
- Ground black pepperto taste
- Vegetable oilto taste
- Eggplant1 kg

COOKING INSTRUCTION 50 MINUTES + 2 HOURS

1. Cut the peel from the eggplant, cut it into circles or along, salt and squeeze it well or put it under the load for a couple of hours to make the glass bitterness.
2. Fry in vegetable oil until they become soft. We put eggplant in a separate bowl.
3. Finely and finely chop the onion and fry it until it becomes transparent and begins to golden.
4. Boil tomatoes over boiling water, peel them, cut, mash and put in a frying pan with onions.
5. Stew on low heat until thickened, 5-7 minutes.
6. Add eggplant, salt, and pepper there.
7. Keep on fire for a couple of minutes - it turns red-violet slurry. Ajapsandal is eaten cold, most often with bread.

Bulgarian eggplant appetizer

ENERGY VALUE PER PORTION
CALORIE CONTENT 270 KCAL
SQUIRRELS 2.1 GRAM
FATS 25.1 GRAM
CARBOHYDRATES 8.2 GRAM
INGREDIENTS
- Eggplant 600 g
- Vinegar 40 ml
- Vegetable oil 100 ml
- Saltto taste
- Chopped parsleyto taste
- Garlic 2 cloves

COOKING INSTRUCTION 30 MINUTES

1. Preheat the grill and fry the eggplant on all sides until soft. Cool slightly and carefully remove the skin. Grind with a knife and transfer to a bowl. Add oil and mash with a wooden spoon until smooth. At the end, add chopped garlic, salt, vinegar, and parsley. Leave on for 15 minutes and mix well again.

Zucchini appetizer with curd cheese

ENERGY VALUE PER PORTION
CALORIE CONTENT 106 KCAL
SQUIRRELS 3,1 GRAM
FATS 7.8 GRAM
CARBOHYDRATES 5.9 GRAM
INGREDIENTS
- Young zucchini 1 piece
- Cucumbers 1 piece
- Mint leaves 5 g
- Garlic 1 clove
- Almette cheese with herbs 150 g
- Cumin (zira) to taste
- Saltto taste
- Freshly ground black pepperto taste

COOKING INSTRUCTION 20 MINUTES

1. Peel and cut the cucumber into small cubes, part of the cucumber can be cut into strips and left for decoration. Chop the garlic, roll up the mint leaves and cut into strips.
2. Zucchini cut into thick slices obliquely and fry them in a grill pan on all sides.
3. Almette mix with mint, cucumber and garlic, salt and pepper.
4. On the slices of zucchini, lay the cheese mass in the form of a wave or make beautiful dumplings.
5. Garnish the appetizer with straws from the cucumber, sprinkle with cumin seeds and freshly ground pepper.

Appetizer with salmon and ham

ENERGY VALUE PER PORTION
CALORIE CONTENT 660 KCAL
SQUIRRELS 44.3 GRAM
FATS 36.7 GRAM
CARBOHYDRATES 41.7 GRAM
INGREDIENTS

- Armenian lavash 2 pieces
- Lightly salted salmon 300 g
- Ham 300 g
- Greensto taste
- Cream cheese 300 g

COOKING INSTRUCTION 15 MINUTES

1. Lavash grease with a thin layer of processed cheese.
2. Cut the salmon into thin slices.
3. Put the salmon on pita bread.
4. Sprinkle with chopped herbs.
5. Lavash with salmon roll into a roll and put for 10-15 minutes in the freezer. Remove and cut into 2-3 cm slices.
6. Also make ham rolls.

Pickled cabbage for a snack

ENERGY VALUE PER PORTION
CALORIE CONTENT 660 KCAL
SQUIRRELS 1.4 GRAM
FATS 46.1 GRAM
CARBOHYDRATES 58.2 GRAM
INGREDIENTS

- carrots
- Garlic 1 head
- Red capsicum 1 piece
- Water 2 cups
- Salt 3 tablespoons
- Sugar 1 cup
- Vegetable oil 1 cup
- Vinegar 1 cup
- White cabbage 2 g

COOKING INSTRUCTION 30 MINUTES + 5 MINUTES

1. Dice the cabbage, grate the carrots on a coarse or Korean grater, chop the garlic and hot pepper into strips
2. Put the food in a pan and mix.
3. Boil the marinade from water, sugar, salt and spices, remove from heat, pour oil and vinegar.
4. Pour the cabbage with a marinade, cover with a plate under a load. Put in a cool place for 2 days.
5. Put the prepared cabbage in banks and store in the refrigerator.

Zucchini spicy appetizer

ENERGY VALUE PER PORTION
CALORIE CONTENT 296 KCAL
SQUIRRELS 8.6 GRAM
FATS1 5.4 GRAM
CARBOHYDRATES 30,4 GRAM
INGREDIENTS

- Zucchini 2 pieces
- Wheat flour 20 g
- Yogurt 250 g
- Vegetable oil 20 ml
- Garlic1 clove
- Dillto taste
- Saltto taste

COOKING INSTRUCTION 25 MINUTES

1. Zucchini cut in half lengthwise and cut in half circles. Roll in lightly salted flour. Fry in hot oil until golden brown. Set aside to cool.
2. Put yogurt in a bowl, squeeze a clove of garlic and salt. Mix well. Put zucchini in a flat dish, fill with sauce. Sprinkle with finely chopped dill before serving.

Pickled onion meat appetizer

ENERGY VALUE PER PORTION
CALORIE CONTENT 134 KCAL
SQUIRRELS 1 GRAM
FATS 0 GRAM
CARBOHYDRATES 34.3 GRAM
INGREDIENTS

- Sweet onion 1 head
- Red onion 1 head
- White wine vinegar 1 cup
- Sugar ½ cup
- Coarse salt 1 tablespoon
- Chives 1 bunch
- Freshly ground black pepperto taste

COOKING INSTRUCTION 30 MINUTES

1. Chop the sweet and red onions finely. Transfer to a bowl and fill with ice water. Close and leave for 30 minutes, 1 time during this time changing the water.
2. Drain the onions and dry well. Transfer to a clean bowl.
3. In a saucepan, mix vinegar, sugar and salt. Bring to a boil, stirring until sugar is dissolved. Pour onion and let cool, stirring occasionally.
4. When the onion with the marinade has cooled, add chopped green onions in small pieces, mix and sprinkle with black pepper.

Swedish bread appetizer

ENERGY VALUE PER PORTION
CALORIE CONTENT 178 KCAL
SQUIRRELS 7.6 GRAM
FATS 5.5 GRAM
CARBOHYDRATES 24.4 GRAM
INGREDIENTS

- Onion 3 heads
- Green apples 3 pieces
- Chicken egg 3 pieces

COOKING INSTRUCTION 15 MINUTES

1. Hard-boiled eggs, cool and clean.
2. Onion, eggs, apples (previously peeled), cut into strips.
3. Season with mayonnaise and add salt to taste.

Stuffed Eggplant Appetizer

ENERGY VALUE PER PORTION
CALORIE CONTENT 434 KCAL
SQUIRRELS 13.7 GRAM
FATS 36,4 GRAM
CARBOHYDRATES 18.1 GRAM
INGREDIENTS

- Eggplant 1 piece
- Olive oil 3 tablespoons
- Tomatoes 3 pieces
- Onion 1 head
- Garlic 1 clove
- Sun-dried tomato paste 2 tablespoons
- Capers 1 tablespoon
- Breadcrumbs 1.5 tablespoons
- Mozzarella Cheese 150 g
- Basil leaves 1 tablespoon
- Grated Parmesan cheese 2 tablespoons
- Saltto taste
- Vegetable oil 2 tablespoons
- Ground black pepperto taste

COOKING INSTRUCTION 30 MINUTES

1. Slice the eggplant along. Grind the rounded pieces for the filling. Spread slices on parchment, grease with olive oil, salt and pepper. Put in the oven, preheated to 180 degrees, for 15 minutes.
2. Put tomatoes in boiling water for a minute, then peel them off. Cut the tomatoes in half, remove the seeds, finely chop the remaining pulp.
3. Prepare the filling. In a large pan, heat a tablespoon of vegetable oil and fry finely chopped onions, chopped pieces of eggplant, which were left for filling, and chopped garlic for 5 minutes. Add chopped tomatoes, chopped basil leaves and tomato paste and cook for another 5 minutes. Put capers, salt, pepper. Allow the mixture to cool.
4. Cut the mozzarella into small pieces, sprinkle them with layers of eggplant, put the filling on top. Roll rolls, wrapping the ends of the slices at the base.
5. Grease the rolls with olive oil. Mix breadcrumbs with grated parmesan, sprinkle rolls with this mixture, put on each roll a basil leaf greased with vegetable oil.
6. Bake for 20 minutes at 180 degrees.

FABBRI Chef Appetizer

INGREDIENTS

- Philadelphia Cheese 250 g
- Lightly salted salmon 300 g
- Strawberry jam 70 g
- Biscofrisa Cookies 200 g
- Red caviar 50 g

COOKING INSTRUCTION 20 MINUTES

1. On each Biscofrisa apply a very thin layer of olive or strawberry jam. Then cover with Philadelphia cheese, put finely chopped salmon, as in the picture. Decorate with red caviar and a small sprig of greens.

Ham and cheese appetizer tartlets

ENERGY VALUE PER PORTION
CALORIE CONTENT 509 KCAL
SQUIRRELS 19.8 GRAM
FATS 38 GRAM
CARBOHYDRATES 18.2 GRAM
INGREDIENTS

- Tartlets1 5 pieces
- Cooked ham 400 g
- 6 eggs
- Cream Cheese 200 g
- Seedless olives 200 g
- Greensto taste

COOKING INSTRUCTION 30 MINUTES

1. Boil, cool and peel the eggs - so that the shell does not burst during cooking, add a tablespoon of vinegar to the water. Grate the eggs on a coarse grater.
2. Finely chop the ham. If you take soft ham, then it excellently rubs on a coarse grater.
3. Finely chop the olives so that they match the size of the grated egg and ham.
4. All of the above should be mixed well.
5. Put the melted cheese into the resulting mass and mix until the cheese is completely dissolved.
6. 3 hours before serving, put on the tartlets, so that the dough has time to soak.

Vegetable snacks with curd cheese

ENERGY VALUE PER PORTION
CALORIE CONTENT 242 KCAL
SQUIRRELS 7.8 GRAM
FATS1 2,4 GRAM
CARBOHYDRATES 26.2 GRAM
INGREDIENTS

- Potato 1 piece
- Turnip 1 piece
- Beets 1 piece
- Radicchio Salad 20 g
- Almette cheese with herbs 30 g
- Cheese "Almette" with porcini mushrooms 30 g
- Almette Cheese with Garlic 30 g
- Almette cheese with Italian tomatoes 30 g
- Parsleyto taste
- Dillto taste
- Honeyto taste
- Sunflower seedsto taste
- Saltto taste
- Freshly ground black pepperto taste

COOKING INSTRUCTION 2 HOURS

1. Thoroughly wash turnips, beets and potatoes and wrap each vegetable separately in foil. In the oven, preheated to 200 degrees, first put the turnips and beets. After 30 minutes, put potatoes to them and leave for another hour.
2. Half the prepared vegetables and put on a board for serving. Have radicchio tear off a couple of beautiful leaves and put them in vegetables. Put on potatoes Almette with porcini mushrooms, on turnips - Almette with herbs, on beets - Almette with garlic, on radicchio - Almette with tomatoes.
3. Garnish with sprigs of dill and parsley leaves. Pour turnips with honey and sprinkle with sunflower seeds. Salt and pepper.

Avocado appetizer with herring and beets

ENERGY VALUE PER PORTION
CALORIE CONTENT 274 KCAL
SQUIRRELS 19.3 GRAM
FATS 17.4 GRAM
CARBOHYDRATES 11.7 GRAM
INGREDIENTS

- Avocado 1 piece
- Canned Herring 1 can
- Tomatoes 1 piece
- Chicken egg 2 pieces
- Red onions ½ heads
- Ground black pepperto taste
- Lemon juiceto taste
- Dillto taste
- Beets1 piece
- Mayonnaiseto taste

COOKING INSTRUCTION 20 MINUTES

1. Option 1: Cut the **INGREDIENTS** into thin plates, lay in layers, lightly greasing with mayonnaise and chopped dill - literally drop by drop.
2. Cool and gently chop into small portions.
3. Option 2: Finely chop and mix all the **INGREDIENTS**. Season with lemon juice and lightly with mayonnaise.
4. Stuff the hard-boiled eggs with the filling.

Summer vegetable snack with zucchini and eggplant

ENERGY VALUE PER PORTION
CALORIE CONTENT 226 KCAL
SQUIRRELS 7 GRAM
FATS 13.1 GRAM
CARBOHYDRATES 22.2 GRAM
INGREDIENTS

- Eggplant 2 pieces
- Zucchini 3 pieces
- Масло cupolive oil
- Cayenne pepper 1 teaspoon
- Garlic 2 cloves
- Coarse saltto taste
- Tomatoes flame 6 pieces
- Red bell pepper 3 pieces
- Chili pepper 2 pieces

COOKING INSTRUCTION 30 MINUTES

1. In a deep frying pan, put the diced eggplant, diced zucchini and chopped
2. Pour water so that it completely covers the vegetables, bring to a boil, cover and cook for 10 minutes.
3. Then add sliced red peppers, finely chopped tomatoes and finely chopped chili peppers. Cook by stirring constantly and not closing the lid until all the liquid has evaporated. Remove from heat and refrigerate.

Fruit appetizer with curd cheese

ENERGY VALUE PER PORTION
CALORIE CONTENT 608 KCAL
SQUIRRELS 6.8 GRAM
FATS 36.8 GRAM
CARBOHYDRATES 63.7 GRAM
INGREDIENTS

- Apple 1 piece
- Nectarines 1 piece
- Pears 1 piece
- Plums 3 pieces
- Butter 50 g
- Sugar 50 g
- Cream cheese Almette 150 g
- Fresh mintto taste
- Honeyto taste
- Dark chocolateto taste
- White chocolateto taste
- Sunflower seedsto taste
- Almond petalsto taste
- Sweet paprikato taste
- Powdered sugarto taste
- Strawberry 7 pieces

COOKING INSTRUCTION 20 MINUTES
1. Remove the core from the apple, wrap in foil and bake in the oven, preheated to 180 degrees, for 20 minutes.
2. Plums rid of seeds. In a small saucepan, heat the sugar, add butter to it. Caramelize in this plum.
3. Strawberries randomly chopped and put in beautiful glasses. Put halves of fruit on plates, put glasses with strawberries in the same place. Put dumplings from Almette on each half. Strawberries should also get their knel.
5. Pour the apple with honey and garnish with fried seeds, sprinkle nectarine with almond petals and paprika. Put caramelized plum on a pear, garnish with almond petals and white chocolate chips. Garnish strawberries with dark chocolate chips and mint leaves.

Mexican Bean and Avocado Appetizer

ENERGY VALUE PER PORTION
CALORIE CONTENT 632 KCAL
SQUIRRELS 18.1 GRAM
FATS 48.1 GRAM
CARBOHYDRATES 35,3 GRAM
INGREDIENTS

- Canned mix of three types of beans 450 g
- Avocado 3 pieces
- Sour cream 1.5 tablespoons
- Taco Spice Mix 1 teaspoon
- Tomatoes 1 piece
- Green onionsto taste
- ½ cupcheddar cheese

COOKING INSTRUCTION 30 MINUTES
1. Place the beans in an even layer on a serving plate.
2. In a bowl, mix mashed avocados, sour cream, and spices. Stir until smooth and lay evenly on the beans.

3. Finely chop the peeled tomatoes and put on top. Sprinkle with grated cheddar and finely chopped green onions.

Appetizer of liver, apples and onions

ENERGY VALUE PER PORTION
CALORIE CONTENT 339 KCAL
SQUIRRELS 21.6 GRAM
FATS 21,2 GRAM
CARBOHYDRATES 16.3 GRAM
INGREDIENTS

- Beef liver 400 g
- Wheat flour 2 tablespoons
- Onion 2 heads
- Apple 2 g
- Saltto taste
- Vegetable oil 4 tablespoons
- Ground black pepperto taste

COOKING INSTRUCTION 25 MINUTES
1. Cut the liver into small slices and beat off a little. Marinate with salt and pepper for 15 minutes.
2. Fry each slice until cooked, pre-roll in flour. Put on a napkin.
3. Onion cut into rings and fry until transparent and golden brown. Put in a separate bowl.
4. From the apples, carefully cut the core, cut into rings and fry in a pan where the onions were fried.
5. Serve as follows - put slices of liver on a pillow of onion, alternating with slices of apples.

Jewish appetizer
ENERGY VALUE PER PORTION
CALORIE CONTENT 406 KCAL
SQUIRRELS 18.3 GRAM
FATS 29.7 GRAM
CARBOHYDRATES 16.9 GRAM
INGREDIENTS

- 5 eggs
- Cream cheese 2 pieces
- Mayonnaise 150 g
- Garlic Feathers 10 g

COOKING INSTRUCTION 15 MINUTES
1. Boil the eggs.
2. Meanwhile, crush the garlic, and grate the cheese.
3. Then finely chop or crush the eggs with a fork.
4. Mix all the **INGREDIENTS**, pour mayonnaise, leave in the refrigerator for about 0.5-1 hours. Then spread on bread and eat like sandwiches.

Kimchi (spicy Korean cabbage appetizer)

ENERGY VALUE PER PORTION
CALORIE CONTENT 95 KCAL
SQUIRRELS 6.4 GRAM
FATS 0.9 GRAM
CARBOHYDRATES 18.2 GRAM
INGREDIENTS

- Water 300 ml
- Chinese cabbage 3 kg
- Onion 1 head
- Chinese pears 1 piece
- Finely chopped garlic 6 tablespoons

- Grated ginger root 1 tablespoon
- Salt 2 tablespoons
- Sugar 1 tablespoon
- Fish sauce 100 ml
- Daikon 300 g
- Green onion 2 bunches
- Rice flour 3 tablespoons
- Kimchi sauce 1 cup

COOKING INSTRUCTION 2 HOURS + 5 MINUTES

1. Rinse the cabbage slightly, cut lengthwise into two parts, cut the stumps. Then dip in water so that water gets between the leaves, this is necessary so that the salt is evenly distributed in the cabbage. Next, take coarse salt and evenly distribute between the leaves. We tear off 3-4 large leaves of cabbage and also salt. They will come in handy later. We put half-heads in a container, fill the water so that they are completely in the water and squeeze on top. Leave to be salted for about 6-8 hours. After about 3 hours, the cabbage must be turned over

2. When the cabbage is salted, it must be washed well under running water, squeezed slightly and put in a colander for 30 minutes.

3. After you wash the cabbage, you need to tear off a large leaf (in the middle of the half) and try on the salt. Naturally, the meatier part of the leaf will be less salty than the end of the leaf. So we will determine how the cabbage salted and how much salt you need to add to the dressing to get a balanced level of salt.

4. Now we are going to refuel. To begin, prepare a rice broth (paste, jelly). Dilute two tablespoons of rice flour (chapsal kara) in 150 ml of cold water, boil the rest of the water and add the diluted flour there. Mix well so that there are no lumps. It should be a paste, just like for wallpaper gluing - the original is to make this broth from one tablespoon of rice with a high content of starch (chap sal) and two cups of water, then cook until a thick paste is obtained. Quite a long procedure, so it is better to do this decoction in a simpler version, as described above.

5. Cut the radish and pear into strips of about 2.5 by 2.5 mm, cut the green onion 5 cm long, and cut the onion in half rings very thinly. Lightly salt the radish, the juice that the radish will give out, then you can drain.

6. Garlic and ginger need to chop (you can through a meat grinder), add the base dressing, fish sauce, sugar, paste. Mix well.

7. The resulting mixture is added to the chopped vegetables and mixed. Let stand for about 30 minutes. Then we try the mixture on the salt and remember how much salt is in the cabbage, add salt if necessary.

8. We put on rubber gloves, and grease each cabbage leaf liberally with the mixture, then you need to fold the leaves tightly back into a half-cup, then take the longest leaf and carefully tie around and put in a container. When everything is laid, take those leaflets that we prepared in advance and cover on top.

9. For a day we leave the container at room temperature (juice should stand out), then put in the refrigerator for three days. Before using kimchi, cut into slices 2.5 cm long.

Mushrooms for a snack

ENERGY VALUE PER PORTION
CALORIE CONTENT 384 KCAL
SQUIRRELS 9.1 GRAM
FATS 28,4 GRAM
CARBOHYDRATES 13,4 GRAM
INGREDIENTS

- 5 tablespoonsolive oil
- Onion 1 head
- Garlic 2 cloves
- 2 carrots
- Dry white wine 275 ml

- Parsley 5 stems
- Bay leaf 1 g
- Fresh mushrooms 750 g
- Tomatoes 2 pieces
- Saltto taste
- Ground black pepperto taste

COOKING INSTRUCTION 30 MINUTES

1. Heat 3 tablespoons of oil in a pan, add finely chopped onions, sliced carrots and cloves of garlic. Cook, stirring, for 5 minutes. Pour in the wine, add two sprigs of parsley and a bay leaf. Salt and pepper and cook for another 5 minutes. Then add mushroom caps and finely chopped tomatoes and cook for another 5 minutes.

2. Remove parsley, bay leaves and garlic. Transfer the mushrooms to a serving dish, sprinkle with the remaining oil and sprinkle with the remaining parsley, which must be finely chopped. Stir well and put in the refrigerator.

Chips with tomatoes and garlic on chips

ENERGY VALUE PER PORTION
CALORIE CONTENT 382 KCAL
SQUIRRELS 9.6 GRAM
FATS 25.6 GRAM
CARBOHYDRATES 23,4 GRAM
INGREDIENTS

- Cheese 100 g
- Tomatoes 300 g
- Greensto taste
- Garlic 2 cloves
- Mayonnaiseto taste
- Potato Chips 100 g
- Olives 1 can
- Black olives 1 can

COOKING INSTRUCTION 10 MINUTES

1. Finely chop the tomatoes. If the tomatoes are very juicy, drain the juice.
2. Finely chop the greens.
3. Grate the cheese on a fine grater.
4. Mix cheese, tomatoes, herbs.
5. Add garlic squeezed through the garlic press.
6. Add mayonnaise, mix.
7. Put the resulting mass on chips.
8. Garnish with olives.

Cod liver appetizer with gherkins

ENERGY VALUE PER PORTION
CALORIE CONTENT 822 KCAL
SQUIRRELS 25.5 GRAM
FATS 57.9 GRAM
CARBOHYDRATES 49.4 GRAM
INGREDIENTS

- Onion 1 piece
- canned cod liver 1 can
- 4 eggs
- Hard cheese 100 g
- Rye baguette 1 piece
- Parsleyto taste

- Gherkins 250 g

COOKING INSTRUCTION 10 MINUTES PRINT

1. Mash the cod liver with a fork.
2. Finely chop the onions, gherkins, eggs.
3. Rub the cheese on a fine grater.

Spicy Watermelon Peel Appetizer

ENERGY VALUE PER PORTION
CALORIE CONTENT 350 KCAL
SQUIRRELS 4.7 GRAM
FATS 1.4 GRAM
CARBOHYDRATES 81.9 GRAM
INGREDIENTS

- Water 3 L
- Watermelon peels 6 cups
- Sugar 1 cup
- Apple cider vinegar 1 cup
- Dry mustard 1.5 tablespoons
- Turmeric 2 teaspoons
- Ground ginger 1.5 teaspoons
- ½ teaspoonsalt
- ½ teaspooncelery seed

COOKING INSTRUCTION 30 MINUTES

1. Cut the watermelon rinds (only the white part, not the green one) into very thin strips and put in a pot of boiling water. Cook for 3 minutes, drain.
2. In a pan, combine sugar, vinegar, mustard, turmeric, ginger, salt, and celery seeds. Bring to a boil, reduce heat and simmer for 2 minutes, stirring occasionally. Add watermelon rinds and cook, without covering, for 30 minutes, until all the liquid has evaporated. Refrigerate and transfer to container.

Smoked Salmon Appetizer

ENERGY VALUE PER PORTION
CALORIE CONTENT 302 KCAL
SQUIRRELS 18.8 GRAM
FATS 20.5 GRAM
CARBOHYDRATES 11.3 GRAM
INGREDIENTS

- Lemon juice 1 tablespoon
- Avocado 1 piece
- Cucumbers 2 pieces
- Celery 1 piece
- Natural yogurt 450 g
- Smoked Salmon 200 g
- Dill 4 tablespoons
- Arugula 1 bunch

COOKING INSTRUCTION 15 MINUTES

1. Cut the cucumber in half and remove the seeds. Cut the cucumber and celery into thin slices.
2. Mash avocados with a fork. Mix with cucumber and celery, add arugula and season with lemon juice.
3. Mix yogurt with chopped dill.
4. Cut the salmon fillet into slices and roll the slices into tubes.
5. Put vegetables at the bottom of the glasses, and yogurt and salmon on top. Garnish with dill.

Pumpkin Appetizer with Pears and Bacon

ENERGY VALUE PER PORTION
CALORIE CONTENT 188 KCAL
SQUIRRELS 4.3 GRAM
FATS 9.7 GRAM
CARBOHYDRATES 25.6 GRAM
INGREDIENTS

- Pumpkin squash 500 g
- Pears 2 pieces
- Extra virgin olive oil 2 teaspoons
- Coarse saltto taste
- Freshly ground black pepperto taste
- Bacon 2 slices
- Water 2 tablespoons
- Brown sugar 1 tablespoon
- Ground chili 1 teaspoon

COOKING INSTRUCTION 35 MINUTES

1. Preheat the oven to 220 degrees.
2. Cut the pears into thin slices along, removing the core and transfer to a bowl.
3. Cut the pumpkin lengthwise into 4 parts, peel the seeds, then thinly cut across the slices. Transfer to pears. Add olive oil, salt and pepper. Stir and place evenly on a baking sheet.
4. Bake until soft, sometimes stirring, for 20–25 minutes.
5. Meanwhile, fry the bacon in a well-heated frying pan until crispy and transfer to a paper towel.
6. In a small saucepan, mix water, sugar and chili until sugar is dissolved.
7. Transfer the pumpkin and pears into a bowl, pour over the syrup and mix.
8. Serve sprinkled with chopped bacon.

Vitello Tonato Appetizer

ENERGY VALUE PER PORTION
CALORIE CONTENT 405 KCAL
SQUIRRELS 29.9 GRAM
FATS 31,2 GRAM
CARBOHYDRATES 0.7 GRAM
INGREDIENTS

- Veal tenderloin 600 g
- Beef broth 1 l
- Canned tuna in its own juice 200 g
- Egg yolk 2 pieces
- Dijon mustard 1 teaspoon
- Sherry vinegar 20 ml
- Olive oil1 50 ml
- Anchovies 25 g
- Lemonto taste
- Garlicto taste
- Saltto taste
- Ground black pepperto taste

COOKING INSTRUCTION 3 HOURS

1. Cut the veal tenderloin from the films into equal pieces about 15 cm in length and wrap in cling film in the manner of sausages. Sausages in a hot beef broth and cook for about 2 hours.
2. In a bowl, beat egg yolks with mustard and slowly pour olive oil into them, continuously whisking the mixture, add vinegar, salt, pepper, a little crushed garlic. In the blender, mix the resulting mayonnaise

with a small amount of broth, anchovies and canned tuna to make a flowing sauce. Season it with lemon juice if you want to make the taste of the sauce live.

3. Cool the veal, cut into thin slices and pour the sauce. Cover with foil, let stand for about half an hour and serve as a cold snack.

Red Bean Spicy Appetizer

ENERGY VALUE PER PORTION
CALORIE CONTENT 929 KCAL
SQUIRRELS 61.8 GRAM
FATS 52 GRAM
CARBOHYDRATES 51.9 GRAM
INGREDIENTS

- Onion1 head
- Ground beef 1 kg
- Garlic 5 cloves
- Beef broth 1 cup
- Ground chili 0.3 cup
- Ground cumin (zira) 1 tablespoon
- Cocoa Powder 1 Tbsp
- Coarse salt 1 teaspoon
- Red canned beans 900 g
- Tomatoes in own juice 410 g
- Apple cider vinegar 1 tablespoon

COOKING INSTRUCTION 45 MINUTES

1. Heat a deep frying pan over medium heat. Add the minced meat and brown for 5 minutes. Add finely chopped onions, mix well and fry for 3-5 minutes. Then add chopped garlic and cook another 1-2 minutes.

2. Pour in the broth slowly, breaking the meatballs. Then add chili, cumin, cocoa and tomatoes. Reduce heat slightly, cover and simmer for 10 minutes.

3. Add beans, vinegar and salt and mix well. Without covering, cook for 10 minutes. Try and add spices and salt to taste. Serve hot with sour cream and corn bread.

Creole Eggplant

ENERGY VALUE PER PORTION
CALORIE CONTENT 421KCAL
SQUIRRELS 7.4 GRAM
FATS 30.7 GRAM
CARBOHYDRATES 31.6 GRAM
INGREDIENTS

- 6 tablespoonsolive oil
- Onion 2 heads
- Garlic4 cloves
- Green bell pepper 1 piece
- Red bell pepper 1 piece
- Eggplant 3 pieces
- Па tablespoonsweet paprika
- Hot pepper ¼ tablespoon
- Ground cumin (zira) 2 teaspoons
- ½ teaspoonbrown sugar
- Saltto taste
- Canned Cherry 800 g
- Freshly ground black pepperto taste

- Chopped parsley 2 tablespoons
- Lime 1 piece

COOKING INSTRUCTION 30 MINUTES

1. Heat 2 tablespoons of olive oil in a pan over medium heat.

2. Add finely chopped onion, finely chopped garlic and peeled and finely chopped bell peppers. Fry, stirring, 3-4 minutes until soft.

3. Meanwhile, in another pan, heat the remaining olive oil and fry the eggplant, sliced in medium cubes, in portions for 4-6 minutes until golden brown. Put a spoon with holes on a plate and keep warm.

4. In a pan with onions and peppers, add both paprika and cumin and fry for about a minute until the aroma is characteristic.

5. Then add canned cherry, sugar, and eggplant. Salt and pepper.

6. Pour 350 ml of water into the pan, bring to a boil, reduce heat and simmer for 15-20 minutes until soft and thick.

7. Sprinkle with parsley and serve with lime slices before serving.

Fast bean snack with cheese crust

ENERGY VALUE PER PORTION
CALORIE CONTENT 344 KCAL
SQUIRRELS 22 GRAM
FATS 11.2 GRAM
CARBOHYDRATES 38.1 GRAM
INGREDIENTS

- Red canned beans 420 g
- ½ cupsalsa sauce
- Canned Pinto Beans 420 g
- Chives 4 stalks
- Cheddar cheese 0.6 cup

COOKING INSTRUCTION 30 MINUTES

1. Preheat the grill in the oven.

2. In a saucepan, mix both beans, salsa sauce and half grated cheese. Put on medium heat and cook until the cheese melts for about 8 minutes.

3. Put the beans in a mold, sprinkle with the remaining cheese and chopped green onions. Grill for 2 minutes until golden brown.

Marinated eggplant and grilled peppers appetizer

ENERGY VALUE PER PORTION
CALORIE CONTENT 170 KCAL
SQUIRRELS 7.7 GRAM
FATS 0.4 GRAM
CARBOHYDRATES 33,4 GRAM
INGREDIENTS

- Eggplant 1 kg
- Dill 1 bunch
- Parsley 1 bunch
- Garlic 1 head
- Water 350 ml
- Salt 1 tablespoon
- Sweet pepper 1 kg
- Sugar 1 tablespoon
- Vinegar 9% 1 tablespoon

COOKING INSTRUCTION 1 HOUR

1. Peppers, peel, rinse, dry, cut into 4 parts - if large, if small - into 2 parts.

Put them on a baking sheet, brush with a vegetable oil brush, bake in the oven at 180-200 degrees until golden brown.

2. Wash, dry eggplants, cut into rings, 1-1.5 cm wide, fry in vegetable oil until golden brown.

3. Finely chop the herbs and garlic.

4. In a convenient wide enameled saucepan (or plastic container), lay the vegetables in layers: eggplant - greens - peppers - greens, etc.

5. Pour vegetables with ready-made chilled marinade. For marinade, add salt, sugar, vinegar to boiled water at room temperature (or bottled) - mix everything until dissolved, and pour vegetables with this marinade.

6. Cool the cooled vegetables with a lid, put in the refrigerator, let it brew for 24 hours, and you can eat.

Asparagus Salmon Appetizer

ENERGY VALUE PER PORTION
CALORIE CONTENT 176 KCAL
SQUIRRELS 11 GRAM
FATS 13,2 GRAM
CARBOHYDRATES 2,5 GRAM
INGREDIENTS

- Green Mini Asparagus 200 g
- Salmon Fillet 200 g
- Saltpinch
- Ground black pepperpinch
- Lemon 1 piece
- 2 tablespoonsolive oil

COOKING INSTRUCTION 15 MINUTES

1. We quickly fry asparagus in olive oil for just a couple of minutes.
2. We take out.
3. Cut the salmon into thin slices.
4. With these slices we wrap 4 asparagus asparagus.
5. Fry again literally for 1.5 minutes on both sides.
6. We remove.
7. Salt, pepper and pour over lemon juice.

Shrimp appetizer with Japanese mayonnaise

ENERGY VALUE PER PORTION
CALORIE CONTENT 360 KCAL
SQUIRRELS 38 GRAM
FATS 19.7 GRAM
CARBOHYDRATES 8.1 GRAM
INGREDIENTS

- Boiled peeled king prawns 20 pieces
- Lime 3 pieces
- Fresh chili pepper 1 piece
- Wasabi pasta 2 teaspoons
- Mayonnaise 100 g
- Chives 2 stalks
- Rice vinegar 2 tablespoons

COOKING INSTRUCTION 20 MINUTES

1. Grate the zest with 2 limes on a fine grater. Transfer to a bowl. Peel the chilli from the seeds and chop finely - shift to the zest. Add the shrimp, mix well, cover with wrap and refrigerate for 1 hour.

2. Meanwhile, in a small bowl, mix mayonnaise, wasabi paste, finely chopped green onions, rice vinegar, grated zest of the remaining lime and 0.5 lime juice. Mix well and transfer to a serving small bowl.

3. Transfer the shrimp to a dish, put Japanese mayonnaise nearby and serve.

Smoked Salmon Appetizer with Fresh Cucumber

ENERGY VALUE PER PORTION
CALORIE CONTENT 895 KCAL
SQUIRRELS 96.7 GRAM
FATS 37,2 GRAM
CARBOHYDRATES 45.3 GRAM
INGREDIENTS

- Sour cream 10%2.5 tablespoons
- Rye bread 16 slices
- Greek yogurt 3 tablespoons
- Dillto taste
- Smoked Salmon 16 pieces
- Cucumbers 16 pieces

COOKING INSTRUCTION 10 MINUTES
1. In a small bowl, mix sour cream and yogurt.
2. Put slices of rye bread on the dish (you can cut circles or squares out of them).
3. On each put a mug of cucumber, a little sauce and a slice of fish. Garnish with dill branches on top.

Quail Egg and Salmon Appetizer

ENERGY VALUE PER PORTION
CALORIE CONTENT 257 KCAL
SQUIRRELS 20.1 GRAM
FATS 20.9 GRAM
CARBOHYDRATES 2 GRAM
INGREDIENTS

- Quail egg 15 pieces
- Salmon1 20 g
- Cucumbers 1 piece
- Cream Cheese 100 g
- Hard cheese 150 g
- Red caviar 50 g
- Greensto taste

COOKING INSTRUCTION 30 MINUTES
1. Cook quail eggs, then clean them.
2. Cut the cheese into plates (1 cm), squeeze the "flowers" out of the plates with a mold. We cut cucumbers with the same form.
3. Put flowers from cheese and cucumbers on a dish, put cream cheese on top. Around the cheese - red caviar.
4. We cut salmon with long and thin plates. Wrap each egg with a salmon plate. We put them at the center of the "flowers".
5. We decorate each canapé with greens and eggs.

Appetizer with pasta, cheese and nutmeg

ENERGY VALUE PER PORTION
CALORIE CONTENT 209 KCAL
SQUIRRELS 8.8 GRAM
FATS 6.6 GRAM
CARBOHYDRATES 25.7 GRAM
INGREDIENTS

- Lemon 1 piece
- Corn starch 2 teaspoons
- Garlic 1 clove

- ½ cupchicken stock
- Kirsch ¼ cup
- Nutmegpinch
- Gruyere cheese ¼ cup
- Swiss cheese 100 g
- Homiti pasta (horns) 230 g
- Breadcrumbs 2 tablespoons
- Green basil 1 bunch
- Ground black pepperpinch

COOKING INSTRUCTION 30 MINUTES

1. Cook the pasta in boiling salted water until almost done. Drain the water.

2. Preheat the oven to 200 degrees. Squeeze the juice of half a lemon in a small bowl and mix with starch.

3. Rub the bottom of the pan with a clove of garlic and, chopping it into pieces, send it there. Add the broth, kirsch and nutmeg. Bring to a boil over medium heat and add grated cheese. Reduce heat slightly and cook until cheese melts, 2-3 minutes. Add the lemon mixture and cook for 30 seconds.

4. Then pour the paste, mix well and put the mass into 8 small molds or coffee cups. Sprinkle with breadcrumbs and place on a baking sheet. Bake for 8-10 minutes. Rearrange on plates, let cool for 4-5 minutes, garnish with basil and sprinkle with black pepper. Pour the remaining lemon juice.

Pineapple rings appetizer

ENERGY VALUE PER PORTION
CALORIE CONTENT 313KCAL
SQUIRRELS 6.8 GRAM
FATS 6 GRAM
CARBOHYDRATES 58.2 GRAM
INGREDIENTS

- Canned pineapple rings8 pieces
- Cheese 100 g
- Mayonnaiseto taste
- Chicken egg 2 pieces
- Crab sticks 100 g
- Green salad 8 slices

COOKING INSTRUCTION 15 MINUTES PRINT

1. Boil the eggs.

2. Cheese, crab sticks (shrimp) and eggs cut into cubes (optional, cheese can be grated on a coarse grater). Mix everything and add mayonnaise.

3. Put lettuce leaves on the pineapple rings (I took an iceberg), put the prepared mixture on top.

Cheese sticks stuffed with cheese

ENERGY VALUE PER PORTION
CALORIE CONTENT 419 KCAL
SQUIRRELS 26,4 GRAM
FATS 25.1 GRAM
CARBOHYDRATES 22 GRAM
INGREDIENTS

- 12 crab sticks
- Hard cheese 300 g
- Green onion feathers1 bunch
- Garlic 3 cloves
- Dill 1 bunch
- Light mayonnaise 200 g

COOKING INSTRUCTION 30 MINUTES

1. Crab sticks untwist. To do this, you need to put all the sticks in turn for a few seconds in very hot water.

2. Grate the cheese on a fine grater, add crushed garlic, 4 tablespoons of mayonnaise, chopped dill, mix everything.

3. Fill ten crab sticks with this filling, place a feather of green onion in the center, fold and lay them in the form of a woodpile (pyramid) on a dish, greasing each layer with a small amount of mayonnaise.

4. Lubricate the whole woodpile on the sides with mayonnaise, grate the remaining two crab sticks on top.

Nut and cheese appetizer

ENERGY VALUE PER PORTION
CALORIE CONTENT 379 KCAL
SQUIRRELS 11,4 GRAM
FATS 33 GRAM
CARBOHYDRATES 10,4 GRAM
INGREDIENTS

- Cream Cheese 160 g
- Crushed walnuts 100 g
- Chicken egg 2 pieces
- Crab sticks 100 g
- Mayonnaise 150 g
- Garlic 1 clove

COOKING INSTRUCTION 30 MINUTES

1. Boil eggs, grate. Cream cheese, too, grate.

2. Fry walnuts and crumble into large crumbs. Finely chop the crab sticks with a knife.

3. Pass the garlic through a garlic squeezer.

4. Use a snack to stuff profiteroles, tartlets or serve on bread.

Warm potato snack with green peas, fried tomatoes and dill

ENERGY VALUE PER PORTION
CALORIE CONTENT 159 KCAL
SQUIRRELS 4.3 GRAM
FATS 8 GRAM
CARBOHYDRATES 20.5 GRAM
INGREDIENTS

- Potato ½ kg
- Cherry Tomatoes 12 pieces
- Red onion 1 piece
- Olive oil GAEA DOP Kalamata extra virgin ⅓ cup
- Frozen Green Peas 1 cup
- Water 4 tablespoons
- Red wine vinegar 3 tablespoons
- Saltto taste
- Ground black pepperto taste
- Dill1 bunch

COOKING INSTRUCTION 35 MINUTES

1. Wash the potatoes well without peeling them. Boil potatoes in salted water until the skin begins to burst and becomes soft (30-35 minutes). Remove from heat, let the potatoes dry and cool slightly.

2. While the potatoes are being boiled, heat 1 tablespoon of olive oil in a pan and sauté the cherry tomatoes until the peel bursts. Salt the tomatoes and remove them from the heat. Passer green peas in the same pan, adding 4 tablespoons of water. Remove and let dry.

3. Peel the warm potatoes and cut them into 4 or 6 pieces. Put on a serving dish, add the tomatoes and green peas, as well as chopped onions. Season the dish with olive oil and wine vinegar, pepper and salt to taste. Add dill and serve immediately.

Hot mushroom appetizer in wine sauce with cheese

ENERGY VALUE PER PORTION
CALORIE CONTENT 1686 KCAL
SQUIRRELS 56 GRAM
FATS 37 GRAM
CARBOHYDRATES 276 GRAM
INGREDIENTS

- Fresh mushrooms 400 g
- Butter 20 g
- Onion 1 head
- White dry wine ½ cup
- Water ½ cup
- Potato starch 3 teaspoons
- Saltto taste
- Edam cheese 80 g
- Freshly ground black pepperto taste
- Fresh thyme 4 stems
- Garlic 1 clove
- French baguette 2 pieces

COOKING INSTRUCTION 25 MINUTES
1. Rinse and peel the mushrooms well. Cut into thin slices.
2. Melt the butter in a pan and add the finely chopped onions and mushrooms. Slightly fry the mushrooms to brown over high heat.
3. Then pour the wine and water. Reduce heat, salt and pepper to taste, add thyme and chopped garlic. Add starch and mix well to thicken the sauce.
4. Put the mushrooms in a refractory form and sprinkle with grated cheese.
5. Preheat the grill in the oven and place mushrooms under it. Bake for about 5 minutes until golden brown. Serve with a crispy baguette.

Avocado appetizer

ENERGY VALUE PER PORTION
CALORIE CONTENT 146 KCAL
SQUIRRELS 1.9 GRAM
FATS 12.6 GRAM
CARBOHYDRATES 7.8 GRAM
INGREDIENTS

- Avocado 1 piece
- Lemon1 piece
- Tomatoes 1 piece
- Garlic 2 cloves
- Saltto taste
- Ground black pepperto taste

COOKING INSTRUCTION 10 MINUTES
1. Peel the avocado, cut it in half, remove the stone. Cut the avocado halves into thin slices and place on a wide, flat dish or large plate.
2. Pour avocado slices with lemon juice, salt, pepper and put a slice of tomato on each slice.

Spicy fetax appetizer

ENERGY VALUE PER PORTION
CALORIE CONTENT 447 KCAL
SQUIRRELS eleven GRAM
FAT S43.5 GRAM
CARBOHYDRATES 3,5 GRAM
INGREDIENTS

- Butter 100 g
- Fetax cheese 200 g
- Chopped dill ½ teaspoon
- Basil 20 g
- Garlic 1 clove
- Walnuts 50 g
- Olives 100 g

COOKING INSTRUCTION 15 MINUTES + 2 HOURS
1. Put walnut, garlic, butter and dill in a blender.
2. Get fetax from the bath and cut into large pieces. Add all the pieces to the blender.
3. Beat all the **INGREDIENTS**.
4. Roll the resulting mass into sausages (you can wrap it in a plastic bag, giving it the desired shape).
5. Put the resulting sausages in the refrigerator for a couple of hours.
6. Cut, garnish with basil, olives and serve.

Red fish appetizer with dill on potato tartlets

ENERGY VALUE PER PORTION
CALORIE CONTENT 202 KCAL
SQUIRRELS 11.1 GRAM
FATS 5.9 GRAM
CARBOHYDRATES 27,2 GRAM
INGREDIENTS

- Yellow onion 150 g
- Potato 500 g
- Chopped dill 1 tablespoon
- Coarse salt to taste
- Freshly ground black pepper to taste
- Lightly salted salmon 120 g
- Egg white 1 piece
- Sour cream 2.5 tablespoons
- Extra virgin olive oil to taste
- Dill to taste

COOKING INSTRUCTION 25 MINUTES
1. Peel onions and potatoes. Grate both on a coarse grater.
2. Preheat the oven to 230 degrees.
3. Squeeze the potatoes and onions lightly. Transfer to a bowl and add dill and protein. Salt and pepper, mix well.
4. Lubricate 2 baking sheets with olive oil.
5. Taking 1 tablespoon of potato mass, blind small pancakes and put on a baking sheet. Put in the oven until golden brown for about 10 minutes. Turn over and return to the oven for another 7 minutes until browned on the other side.
6. Put the pancakes on the dish. Put a piece of fish on top and garnish with sour cream. Garnish with sprigs of dill and serve.

Sweet and Sour Zucchini Appetizer

ENERGY VALUE PER PORTION
CALORIE CONTENT 260 KCAL
SQUIRRELS 5. 1 GRAM
FATS14,4GRAM
CARBOHYDRATES 32.3 GRAM
INGREDIENTS

- Zucchini 4 pieces
- Honey 7.5 tablespoons
- White wine vinegar ½ cup
- Green bell pepper ¼ pieces
- Celery stalk ¼ pieces
- Vegetable oil 0.3 cups
- Onion 20 g
- Salt1 teaspoon
- Ground black pepper 1 teaspoon

COOKING INSTRUCTION 30 MINUTES

1. In a large bowl, mix the finely chopped zucchini, honey, vinegar, vegetable oil, finely chopped green pepper, finely chopped celery, finely chopped onion, salt and pepper. Mix well, cover with foil and send overnight in the refrigerator.
2. The next day, drain excess moisture and serve.

Eggplant cold appetizer

ENERGY VALUE PER PORTION
CALORIE CONTENT 58 KCAL
SQUIRRELS 2.7 GRAM
FATS 0.3 GRAM
CARBOHYDRATES 11.2 GRAM
INGREDIENTS

- Eggplant 4 pieces
- Onion 4 g
- Tomatoes 5 pieces
- Cilantro 50 g
- Red bell pepper 4 pieces
- Garlic 3 cloves
- Tomato paste 2 tablespoons

COOKING INSTRUCTION 1 HOUR

1. Cut eggplant into large slices.
2. We salt so that bitterness will leave, and leave for half an hour.
3. Cut the onion into half rings.
4. Passage to golden color.
5. Scald tomatoes with boiling water so that it is easy to peel.
6. Bulgarian pepper bake in the oven for 40 minutes.

Appetizer with herring, beetroot pesto and walnuts

ENERGY VALUE PER PORTION
CALORIE CONTENT 524 KCAL
SQUIRRELS 19,2 GRAM
FATS 41 GRAM
CARBOHYDRATES 22.2 GRAM
INGREDIENTS

- Norwegian slightly salted herring 1 piece

- Beets 3 pieces
- Garlic 3 cloves
- Walnuts 100 g
- Dill ½ beam
- Parsley ½ bunch
- Olive oil 3 tablespoons
- Sugar 1 teaspoon
- Saltto taste
- Ground black pepperto taste

COOKING INSTRUCTION 40 MINUTES PRINT

1. Peel herring, disassemble on a fillet and cut into slices.
2. Boil the beets, cool.
3. Peel boiled beets, cut into small cubes.
4. Fry nuts in a dry hot frying pan for 2-3 minutes.
5. Chop greens and garlic.
6. Put beets, nuts and greens with garlic in a cup, chop with a blender.
7. Add lemon juice, oil, sugar, salt and pepper. Mix well.
8. Put a beetroot pesto on a slice of black bread, on top 1-2 slices of herring fillet.
9. Garnish with a slice of lemon and herbs.

Alaska pollock fillet snack

ENERGY VALUE PER PORTION
CALORIE CONTENT 254 KCAL
SQUIRRELS 35.5 GRAM
FATS 11.3 GRAM
CARBOHYDRATES 3,5 GRAM
INGREDIENTS
- Pollock fillet 4 pieces
- Black peppercorns 1 teaspoon
- Allspice Peas1 teaspoon
- Sunflower oilto taste
- Dill 1 bunch
- Balsamic vinegarto taste
- Mayonnaise 3 tablespoons
- 4 pickled cucumbers
- Saltto taste

COOKING INSTRUCTION 25 MINUTES PRINT

1. Chop 2 types of peppers
2. Cut the fish fillet into small portions
3. Pickle pieces of fish in a mixture of peppers, salt, slightly sprinkle with balsamic vinegar
4. Heat sunflower oil in a pan
5. Fry the pieces of fish in a pan.
6. While the fish is fried, finely chop the dill and pickled cucumbers. Mix with mayonnaise
7. Put the pieces of fish, garnish with dill, add the sauce.

Soups

Gazpacho soup with watermelon

Preparation: 25 minutes.
Serves: 4
INGREDIENTS:
- Ice cubes – 1 cup
- Seedless watermelon – 6 oz.
- Juiced lime - 1
- Sherry vinegar – 1 tspn
- Peeled and cubed tomatoes – 4
- Garlic clove - 1
- Seeded red pepper - 1
- Shallot - 1
- Pepper and salt to taste

Directions:
1. In a blender, mix all the **INGREDIENTS:**.
2. Make it creamy and smooth by pulsing it. But add pepper and salt first.
3. Serve it chilled in a bowl.

Gorgeous Kale Soup made with white bean
Cooking and preparation: 1 hour.
Serves: 8
INGREDIENTS:
- Drained white beans – 1 can
- Shredded kale – 1 bunch
- Chopped shallot – 1
- Water – 6 cups
- Chopped garlic cloves - 2
- Diced carrots - 2
- Lemon juice – 2 tbsps
- Diced tomatoes – 1 can
- Chopped red pepper - 1
- Vegetable stock – 2 cups
- Pepper and salt to taste
- Olive oil – 2 tbsps
- Diced celery stalk - 1

Directions:
1. Stir in a soup pot celery, garlic, carrots, shallot, red pepper and heated oil. Soften it by cooking for 2 minutes.
2. Add other **INGREDIENTS:** and season with pepper and salt.
3. On low heat, cook the soup for 30 minutes.
4. Enjoy the soup as you serve it chill or warm.

Tomato spiced Haddock Soup recipe

Cooking and preparation: 30 minutes.
Serves: 6
INGREDIENTS:
- Peeled and diced tomatoes - 4
- Sherry vinegar – 1 tspn

- Bay leaf - 1
- Chopped shallot - 1
- Diced celery stalk - 1
- Water – 2 cups
- Cubed haddock fillets – 4
- Minced garlic cloves - 2
- Thyme sprig - 1
- Dried oregano – ½ tspn
- Olive oil – 2 tbsps.
- Pepper and salt to taste
- Vegetable stock – 2 cups

Directions:
1. Stir in a soup pot garlic, shallot and heated oil. Then make it fragrant by cooking it for 2 minutes.
2. Add vinegar, oregano, stock, celery, thyme, tomatoes, water, bay leaf, pepper and salt.
3. Also add haddock after cooking for 15 minutes and with a lid, cover the pot.
4. On low hear, cook for extra 10 minutes. Serve it fresh and warm.

Fast Delicious Avocado Soup

Preparation: 20 minutes
Serves: 6
INGREDIENTS:
- Mint leaves – 2
- Peeled cucumbers – 4
- Chopped shallot - 1
- Water – 1 cup
- Plain yogurt – ½ cup
- Lemon juice – 2 tbsps.
- Fresh basil leaves – 2
- Garlic cloves - 2
- Extra virgin olive oil – 2 tbsps.
- Peeled and pitted avocados - 2
- Pepper and salt to taste

Directions:
1. In a blender, add and mix all the **INGREDIENTS:**. Make it creamy and smooth by pulsing it after the addition of pepper and salt.
2. Serve the soup immediately after pouring into bowls.

Delicious Mixed Barley Soup

Preparation and cooking: 1 hour
Serves: 8
INGREDIENTS:
- Barley – ¼ cup
- Chopped shallots – 2
- Extra virgin olive oil – 2 tbsps.
- Cubed zucchini – 1
- Chopped garlic cloves - 2
- Diced carrots - 2
- Cored and diced yellow bell pepper – 1
- Diced and cored red bell pepper - 1

- Peeled and cubed potatoes - 2
- Drained canned corn – ½ cup
- Diced tomatoes – 1 can
- Bay leaf - 1
- Dried tarragon – ½ tsp.
- Water – 7 cups
- Vegetable stock – 2 cups
- Pepper and salt to taste

Directions:
1. Make it fragrant by stirring garlic, shallots and heated oil in a soup pot for 2 minutes. then add other INGREDIENTS:.
2. On low heat, cook for 30 minutes after seasoning with pepper and salt.
3. Freshly serve the soup warm.

Whitish Bean Soup delicacy

Cooking and preparation: 50 minutes
Serves: 8
INGREDIENTS:
- Baby spinach – 2 cups
- Diced carrots – 2
- Chopped shallots – 2
- Sliced celery stalks - 2
- Chopped garlic cloves – 2
- Cored and diced yellow bell peppers - 2
- Drained white beans – 1 can
- Thyme sprig – 1
- Cubed zucchini - 1
- Rosemary sprig - 1
- Chicken stock – 2 cups
- Diced tomatoes – 1 can
- Water – 6 cups
- Olive oil – 2 tbsps.
- Pepper and salt to taste

Directions:
1. In a soup pot, heat the oil and stir in the peppers, shallots, garlic, carrots and celery.
2. Add other INGREDIENTS: after cooking for 10 minutes on low heat and season with pepper and salt.
3. Allow soup to cook for extra 20 minutes.
4. Freshly serve the soup warm.

Special Delicious Veggie Soup

Preparation and cooking: 1 hour
Serves: 8
INGREDIENTS:
- Cored and diced yellow bell pepper - 1
- Sliced celery stalk – 1
- Chopped garlic clove - 1
- Chopped sweet onion – 1
- Peeled and cubed pounds potatoes – 1 ½
- Vegetable stock – 2 cups

- Water – 7 cups
- Olive oil – 2 tbsps.
- Greek yogurt for serving – ½ cup
- Pepper and salt to taste
- Diced carrots - 2

Directions:
1. Stir in a soup pot carrots, onion, pepper, celery, garlic and heated oil.
2. Add salt, potatoes, water, pepper and stock after cooking for 5 minutes.
3. On low heat, cook the soup for 20 minutes. Remove from heat when the soup is done. Then pour it into serving bowls.
4. Add Greek yogurt when serving.

One Hour Fennel Soup

Servings 6
Preparation and Cooking Time 1 hour
INGREDIENTS:
- Leek - 1, sliced
- Garlic cloves - 3, chopped
- Olive oil - 2 tbsp.
- Shallot - 1, chopped
- Stalk of celery – 1, diced
- Carrot - 1, diced
- Fennel bulb - 1, sliced
- Vegetable stock - 2 cups
- Potato - 1, peeled and cubed
- Tomatoes - 2, peeled and diced
- Harissa powder - ¼ tsp.
- Lemon juice - 1 tbsp.
- Cumin powder - ¼ tsp.
- Water - 1 cup
- Salt and pepper - to taste
- Thyme - 1 sprig

Directions:
1. Add olive oil to pot and heat.
2. After oil is heated, add carrot, celery, leek, fennel, shallot and garlic and cook for 5 minutes.
3. Add in the rest of the INGREDIENTS: above (salt and pepper to suit your taste) and cook for an additional few minutes until vegetables are well cooked.
4. This soup is delicious warm or chilled.

Broccoli Cheese Soup

Servings 6
Preparation and Cooking Time 35 minutes
INGREDIENTS:
- Green chili - 1, chopped
- Extra virgin olive oil - 2 tbsp.
- Garlic cloves - 2, chopped
- Shallot - 1, chopped
- Dried oregano - ½ tsp.
- Water - 1 cup
- Broccoli - 1 ½ lbs., cut into florets

- Salt and pepper - to taste
- Dried basil - ½ tsp.
- Vegetable stock - 2 cups
- Camembert cheese - 4 oz., crumbled
- Heavy cream - ¼ cup

Directions:
1. Olive oil should be heated in a pot and then add green chili, garlic and shallots, cooking for 2 minutes.
2. After 2 minutes, stir in stock, water, oregano, basil, broccoli and salt and pepper to taste.
3. Cook for an additional 10 minutes.
4. Remove from heat and puree in an immersion blender, stirring in cream.
5. Top the soup with camembert cheese and serve.

White Bean Vegetable Soup

Servings 6
Preparation and Cooking Time 40 minutes
INGREDIENTS:
- Garlic cloves - 2, chopped
- Carrots - 2, diced
- Olive oil - 2 tbsp.
- Shallots - 2, sliced
- Celery - 2 stalks, sliced
- Chicken stock - 4 cups
- Water - 2 cups
- Rosemary - 1 sprig
- White beans - 2 cans, drained
- Salt and pepper - to taste

Directions:
1. Pour olive oil in a pot and heat.
2. Then add in garlic and shallots, cooking for approximately 5 minutes.
3. Mix in water, stock, rosemary, carrots, beans and celery and season with salt and pepper to suit your taste.
4. Cook an additional 15 minutes. Serve up soup while fresh.

Soup of the Sea

Servings 8
Preparation and Cooking Time 50 minutes
INGREDIENTS:
- Flounder fillets - 2, cubed
- Fresh mussels - 1 lb., cleaned and rinsed
- Cod fillets - 2, cubed
- Shallots - 2, chopped
- Olive oil - 3 tbsp.
- Garlic cloves - 2, chopped
- Carrots - 2, sliced
- Tomatoes - 2, sliced
- Celery – 1 stalk, sliced
- Red bell peppers 2, cored and sliced
- Tomatoes - 1 cup, diced
- Water - 2 cups

- Dry white wine - 1 cup
- Tomato juice - ½ cup
- Chicken stock - 2 cups
- Bay leaf - 1 leaf
- Salt and pepper - to taste
- Thyme - 1 sprig

Directions:
1. Olive oil should be heated in a pot and then mix in bell peppers, carrots, garlic, celery and shallots.
2. After cooking for 10 minutes, mix in tomato juice, water, stock, wine and tomatoes and cook an additional 15 minutes.
3. Add flounder, mussels, bay leaf, thyme and cod to the pot.
4. Season with salt and pepper and cook for a final 5 minutes. Enjoy!

Creamy Butternut Squash Soup

Servings: 4
Preparation time: 12 minute
Cooking time: 30minutes
INGREDIENTS:
- 2 teaspoon black pepper.
- 4 cans unsalted herbal soup.
- 2 cans chopped butternut squash
- 3 tablespoon olives oil.
- 1 teaspoon salt.
- 2 teaspoons dried thyme.
- 2 celery stalk. chopped
- 2 chopped carrots.

Directions:
1. First Heat the olive oil till it simmers.
2. Increase the sliced onion carrot celery. **Directions:** to 5 to 7 minutes. till the vegetables begin to brown.
3. Mix the soup squash thyme sea salt and pepper.Bring to simmer then decrease heat to minimum. Simmer to 20 minutes till the squash is lenient.
4. Squash the broth using an immersion mixer food processor blender.

Tasty Chicken and Vegetable Soup

Servings: 8
Preparation time: 10 minutes
Cooking time: 20 minutes
INGREDIENTS:
- 1 (14-ounce) crushed tomatoes undrained
- 1 fennel bulb,
- 1 chopped onion.
- 1 tablespoon dried Italian seasoning
- 1 pinch salt.
- 1/2 pinch black pepper.
- 13 ounces boneless skinless sliced chicken breast.
- 2 carrots chopped
- 2 tablespoons olive oil.
- 3 chopped zucchini.

- 6 minced garlic cloves.
- 6 cups unsalted chicken broth

Directions:
1. Put large bowl over high heat until the olive oil begin to simmer. Then add chicken and cooki for about 6 minutes.
2. Remove the chicken from bowl with the help of spoon and put it aside.
3. Add carrots onion red bell pepper and fennel to the oil remaining in the pot. **Directions:** for about 5 minutes stirring occasionally.
4. Add garlic and **Directions:** for 30 seconds stirring constantly.
5. Stir in the broth tomatoes zucchini. Italian seasoning sea salt and pepper. Bring to a boil stirring occasionally. Reduce the heat and simmer for about 5 minutes more.
6. Return the chicken to the pot. **Directions:** for 1 minute more until the chicken heats through. Serve immediately.

Peas and Orzo Soup

Preparation time: 10 minutes
Cooking time: 10 minutes
Servings: 4
INGREDIENTS:
- ½ cup orzo
- 6 cups chicken soup
- 1 and ½ cups cheddar, shredded
- Salt and black pepper to the taste
- 2 teaspoons oregano, dried
- ¼ cup yellow onion, chopped
- 3 cups baby spinach
- 2 tablespoons lime juice
- ½ cup peas

Directions:
1. Heat up a pot with the soup over medium heat, add the orzo and the rest of the **INGREDIENTS** except the cheese, bring to a simmer and cook for 10 minutes.
2. Add the cheese, stir, divide into bowls and serve.

Nutrition Value: calories 360, fat 10.2, fiber 4.7, carbs 43.3, protein 22.3

Rosemary Kale Soup

Preparation time: 10 minutes
Cooking time: 25 minutes
Servings: 4
INGREDIENTS:
- 1 pound kale, torn
- Salt and black pepper to the taste
- 3 tablespoons olive oil
- 1 celery stalk, chopped
- 1 yellow onion, chopped
- 1 carrot, chopped
- 14 ounces canned tomatoes, chopped
- 2 tablespoons rosemary, chopped
- 4 cups veggie stock

Directions:
1. Heat up a pot with the oil over medium heat, add the onion, celery and the carrot and sauté for 5 minutes.
2. Add the rest of the **INGREDIENTS**, simmer the soup over medium heat for 20 minutes, ladle into bowls and serve.

Nutrition Value: calories 192, fat 8.3, fiber 4.5, carbs 12.3, protein 4.5

Chili Watermelon Soup

Preparation time: 4 hours
Cooking time: 0 minutes
Servings: 4
INGREDIENTS:
- 2 pounds watermelon, peeled and cubed
- ½ teaspoon chipotle chili powder
- 2 tablespoons olive oil
- A pinch of salt and white pepper
- 1 tomato, chopped
- 1 shallot, chopped
- ¼ cup cilantro, chopped
- 1 small cucumber, chopped
- 2 tablespoons lemon juice
- ½ tablespoon red wine vinegar

Directions:
1. In a blender, combine the watermelon with the chili powder, the oil and the rest of the **INGREDIENTS** except the vinegar and the lemon juice, pulse well, and divide into bowls.
2. Top each serving with lemon juice and vinegar and serve.

Nutrition Value: calories 120, fat 4.5, fiber 3.4, carbs 12, protein 2.3

Shrimp Soup

Preparation time: 10 minutes
Cooking time: 5 minutes
Servings: 6
INGREDIENTS:
- 1 cucumber, chopped
- 3 cups tomato juicc
- 3 roasted red peppers, chopped
- 3 tablespoons olive oil
- 2 tablespoons balsamic vinegar
- 1 garlic clove, minced
- Salt and black pepper to the taste
- ½ teaspoon cumin, ground
- 1 pounds shrimp, peeled and deveined
- 1 teaspoon thyme, chopped

Directions:
1. In your blender, mix cucumber with tomato juice, red peppers, 2 tablespoons oil, the vinegar, cumin, salt, pepper and the garlic, pulse well, transfer to a bowl and keep in the fridge for 10 minutes.
2. Heat up a pot with the rest of the oil over medium heat, add the shrimp, salt, pepper and the thyme and cook for 2 minutes on each side.
3. Divide cold soup into bowls, top with the shrimp and serve.

Nutrition Value: calories 263, fat 11.1, fiber 2.4, carbs 12.5, protein 6.32

Turmeric Chard Soup

Preparation time: 10 minutes
Cooking time: 40 minutes
Servings: 6
INGREDIENTS:

- 2 tablespoons olive oil
- 1 pound chard, chopped
- 1 teaspoon coriander seeds, ground
- 2 teaspoons mustard seeds
- 2 teaspoons garlic, minced
- 1 tablespoon ginger, grated
- ¼ teaspoon cardamom, ground
- ¼ teaspoon turmeric powder
- 1 yellow onion, chopped
- ¾ cup rhubarb, sliced
- Salt and black pepper to the taste
- 5 cups water
- 3 tablespoons cilantro, chopped
- 6 tablespoons yogurt

1. **Directions:**
2. Heat up a pan with the oil over medium heat, add the coriander, mustard seeds, garlic, ginger, cardamom, turmeric and the onion, stir and sauté for 5 minutes.
3. Add the rest of the **INGREDIENTS** except the cilantro and the yogurt, bring to a simmer and cook for 20 minutes.
4. Divide the soup into bowls, top each serving with cilantro and yogurt and serve.

Nutrition Value: calories 189, fat 8.3, fiber 3.4, carbs 11.7, protein 4.5

Garbanzo and Lentil Soup

Serves: 8
Cooking time: 90 minutes
INGREDIENTS:

- 1 14.5-oz can petite diced tomatoes, undrained
- 2 15-oz cans Garbanzo beans, rinsed and drained
- 1 cup lentils
- 6 cups vegetable broth
- ¼ tsp ground cayenne pepper
- ½ tsp ground cumin
- 1 tsp turmeric
- 1 tsp garam masala
- 1 tsp minced garlic
- 2 tsp grated fresh ginger
- 1 cup diced carrots
- 1 cup chopped celery
- 2 onions, chopped

Directions for Cooking:

1. On medium high fire, place a heavy bottomed large pot and grease with cooking spray.
2. Add onions and sauté until tender, around three to four minutes.
3. Add celery and carrots. Cook for another five minutes.

4. Add cayenne pepper, cumin, turmeric, ginger, garam masala and garlic, cook for half a minute.
5. Add diced tomatoes, garbanzo beans, lentils and vegetable broth. Bring to a boil.
6. Once boiling, slow fire to a simmer and cook while covered for 90 minutes. Occasionally stir soup.
7. If you want a thicker and creamier soup, you can puree ½ of the pot's content and mix in.
8. Once lentils are soft, turn off fire and serve.

Nutrition Information: Calories per serving: 196; Protein: 10.1g; Carbs: 33.3g; Fat: 3.6g

Kidney and Black Bean Chicken Soup

Serves: 10
Cooking time: 7 hours
INGREDIENTS:

- 2 chicken breasts fillets, skinless, cut into 1-inch cubes
- ½ cup freshly chopped cilantro
- Salt to taste
- ½ tsp black pepper
- ½ tsp cayenne pepper
- 1 tsp cumin
- 1 tbsp chili powder
- Juice from 1 lime
- 1 cup fresh or frozen corn kernels
- 2 ½ cups chicken broth, low sodium, fat free
- 1 14.5-oz can diced tomatoes
- 1 4.5-oz can diced green chili peppers
- 1 15-oz can kidney beans, rinsed and drained
- 1 15-oz can black beans, rinsed and drained
- 1 clove garlic, minced
- ½ cup diced onion

Directions for Cooking:

1. In slow cooker, add all **INGREDIENTS**.
2. Cover and cook on low settings for six to eight hours.
3. When done, transfer to serving bowls and enjoy.

Nutrition Information: Calories per serving: 192; Protein: 20.0g; Carbs: 21.0g; Fat: 12.8g

Moroccan Delicious Seafood Soup

INGREDIENTS:

- Thinly sliced red onion – 1
- Harissa – 1 tablespoon
- Fish stock – 500ml
- Peeled and chopped tomatoes – 2
- Grounded ginger – ½ teaspoon
- Fish preferably snapper or cod – 1 kg
- Prawns – 8
- Lemon – 1
- Celery stalk – 1
- Coriander seeds – 1 tablespoon
- Olive Oil – 2 tablespoon
- Cleaned and sliced into rings – 250g squid
- Chopped flat leaf parsley – 3 tablespoon

Directions:

1. Heat the oil in a saucepan and fry the onion.
2. Add up the coriander, ginger, harissa and parsley and get it cooked for 5 minutes.
3. Add salt and the grounded black pepper and stir continuously.
4. Add in the tomatoes and cook for 5 minutes before adding the stock.
5. Mix in the seafood and cook for 15 minutes until it's fully cooked.
6. Add lemon juice to the ladle in the soup bowls. Get it served with bread and extra dollop.

Fish Soup with Soft Olives and Wine

INGREDIENTS:

- Coarsely chopped onion - 1
- Large cloves garlic – 2
- Bay leaf – 1
- Chilli flakes – ¼ teaspoon
- Peeled and deveined prawns – 375g
- Thick slices of toasted bread – 4
- Fish stock – 4 cups
- Calamari – 375g
- Stalk Celery with leaves – 1
- Ling fillets – 400g
- Salt – ¾ teaspoon
- Extra virgin olive oil- 1 tablespoon
- Dry white wine – ½ cup
- Black mussels – 375g

Directions:

1. Add some oil in a heavy based saucepan and heat moderately. Add onions and cook for 5 minutes until it gets soft.
2. Pour in the garlic and the calamari, stir it for 5 minutes, after then you can remove the slotted spoon set aside.
3. Add some wine to the saucepan and cook for 3 minutes. In another separate saucepan, and boil under a moderate heat for 5 minutes.
4. Put away the ones that didn't open and sieve away with a damp paper towel.
5. Strain off the liquid from the mussels and add to the soup mixture. Pour slowly the celery, Olives, bay leaf, salt, chilli and 2 tablespoons parsley and boil for 3 minutes.
6. Mix in the prawns, mussels and reserved calamari and boil for 3 minutes.
7. Put the toast in heated bowls, and served the soup sprinkled with the remaining parcel.

Pasta Seafood Soup

Preparation time:
20 minutes
Cooking time: 20 minutes
Servings: 4
INGREDIENTS:

- Pasta-1/3 cup
- Saffron threads-1pinch
- Tomatoes, chopped coarsely-5
- Red chilies, seeded-2
- Mixed herbs, chopped-1/2 cup
- Olive oil-1tablespoon
- Vegetable stock-3cup

- Onion, diced-1
- White wine-1/2cup
- Garlic cloves, sliced-2
- Mixed seafood-2lb
- Crusty bread, to serve
- Hot water-2tablespoon

Directions:
1. In a bowl add some hot water and add the saffron. Stir and set aside for now.
2. In a pan heat the oil and add the garlic cloves and onion. Cook for 3 minutes and add the tomatoes.
3. Add the red chilies and vegetable stock. Mix well and let it come to a boil.
4. Run the mix through a strainer and remove any solids. Return to heat and add the pasta, saffron mix and cook for 10 minutes.
5. Add salt and pepper and mix well. In another pan boil the white wine.
6. Add the seafood mix and cook for about 5 minutes. Serve the seafood into individual bowls.
7. Pour the tomato mix into each bowls.
8. Serve with bread.

Mediterranean soup

INGREDIENTS
- Fish fillet (pollock, haddock, cod) - 500 g
- Tomato - 450 g
- Rice - 200 g
- Broth (fish, vegetable or water) - 200 ml
- Dry white wine - 200 ml
- Almonds (chopped) - 2 tbsp. l
- Onion - 2 pcs.
- Petiole celery - 2 pcs.
- Thyme (twigs or 1/2 tsp. Dry thyme) - 2
- Bay leaf - 2 pcs.
- Olive oil - 3 tbsp. l

Directions
1. Chop the onion and fry in oil with almonds.
2. Add wine, broth, chopped tomatoes, sliced celery and bay leaf.
3. Salt and pepper. Cook over low heat under a lid for about 15 minutes.
4. If using fresh thyme, tear off the leaves and put in the broth 5 minutes before being ready
5. Rinse the fish, dry and cut into portions. Salt and pepper
6. Boil rice.
7. Add fish to the broth,
8. Dry thyme, if used, and simmer for about 10 minutes under a lid over low heat.
9. Put a slide of rice on a plate, carefully pour the soup around and lay out the pieces of fish. Garnish with greens.

seafood, fish and rice noodle soup

INGREDIENTS ON
8 PORTION
- The main parsley tastechives
- Taste rice noodles
- 60 gwater
- Taste salt

- taste ground black pepper
- taste Bay leaf
- 2 pcs. canned tomatoes in their own juice
- ½ cans frozen squids
- 100 g white fillet fish
- 150 g carrot
- 1 PC. garlic
- 3 cloves olive oil
- 4 tbsp. L bell pepper red
- 1 PC. chilli
- 1 PC. potatoes
- 3 pcs. tiger prawns
- 200 g frozen shrimp

Directions

1. Boil shrimp and squid in salted water with black peppercorns and bay leaf. Cool and peel the shrimp from the shell. Strain broth from seafood through a sieve and save, we still need it.
2. Cut the carrots into circles.
3. Peel the garlic.
4. With a saucepan in which you will cook the soup, pour olive oil. Put carrots in the heated oil and, through the press, garlic.
5. Add it to the pan to the carrots and garlic.
6. Peel the chili peppers (I have yellow) and chop finely.
7. Add chili peppers to vegetables.
8. Peel and cut the potatoes into cubes.
9. Pour the vegetables with strained seafood broth. If it is not enough, then add more boiled water. Dip the potatoes there and cook for 8-10 minutes.
10. Add half a can of tomato to the soup (I have chopped, in my own juice). Let it boil.
11. Wash the white fish fillet (I have herring), dry it with a paper towel.
12. Cut the fish and add to the soup. Let it boil for a couple of minutes.
13. Cut the squids in half and add to the soup.
14. Add shrimp at the end. Let the soup boil and remove the pan from the stove.
15. The soup is almost ready. It remains to cook the noodles.
16. Break rice noodles into pieces.
17. Pour boiling water, cover and leave according to the instructions (with me) for 3 minutes.
18. Then drain the water and rinse the noodles in a colander with cold water.
19. You can add noodles to the soup, or you can put it into soup bowls and pour the soup on top. Do as you prefer.
20. Sprinkle soup with chives and garnish with parsley. Bon Appetit!

Reddish Mediterranean Bean Soup

Preparation time: 45 minutes
Servings: 8
INGREDIENTS:

- Chopped red onions - 2
- Diced celery stalks - 2
- Cored and diced red bell peppers - 2
- Diced carrots - 2
- Drained and rinsed red beans – 2 cans
- Diced tomatoes – 1 can
- Tomato paste – 2 tbsps.

- Vegetable stock – 2 cups
- Water – 7 cups
- Thyme sprig – 1
- Olive oil – 2 tbsps.
- Rosemary sprig - 1
- Chopped parsley (for serving)
- Pepper and salt to taste

Directions:
1. Stir in a soup of pot celery, carrots, red onions, bell peppers and heated oil.
2. Add other **INGREDIENTS:** after cooking for 5 minutes.
3. Then season with pepper and salt.
4. On low heat, stir in chopped parsley after cooking for 25 minutes. Freshly serve the soup when it's warm.

Cauliflower Soup With Cream

Preparation time: 35 minutes
Servings: 6
INGREDIENTS:
- Chopped garlic cloves - 2
- Chicken stock – 2 cups
- Large head cauliflower – 1 (cut into florets)
- Pepper and salt to taste
- Rosemary sprig – 1
- Chopped shallot - 1
- Heavy cream – ½ cup
- Olive oil – 2 tbsps.
- Feta cheese for serving – 3 oz.

Directions:
1. Stir in a soup pot garlic, shallow and heated oil.
2. Add pepper, cauliflower, rosemary sprig, salt and stock after cooking for 2 minutes.
3. On low heat, remove the rosemary after cooking for 15 minutes and stir in the cream.
4. Use immersion blender to puree the soup and serve the soup chilled or warm, top it with crumbled feta cheese.

Very Veggie Soup

Servings 8
Preparation time: 1 hour
INGREDIENTS:
- Olive oil - 2 tbsp.
- Stalk of celery - 1, sliced
- Garlic clove - 1, chopped
- Sweet onion - 1, chopped
- Small fennel bulb - 1, sliced
- Carrot - 1, diced
- Potatoes - 2, peeled and cubed
- Leek - 1, sliced
- Tomatoes - 2, peeled and diced
- Chicken stock - 4 cups
- Water - 4 cups
- Tomato paste - 2 tbsp.

- Salt and pepper - to taste

Directions:
1. Pour olive oil into a pot and heat.
2. Add in celery, garlic, onion, fennel, carrot and leek, stirring well.
3. After cooking for 5 minutes you can stir in water, chicken stock and potatoes.
4. Add salt and pepper to suit your personal taste.
5. Set heat to low and cook for 25 minutes. Soup is hot and ready to eat.

Sausage and Multi Bean Minestrone

Servings 10
Preparation time: 1 hour
INGREDIENTS:
- Chicken sausage - 2, sliced
- Green bell pepper - 1, cored and diced
- Olive oil - 2 tbsp.
- Shallots - 2, chopped
- Garlic clove - 1, chopped
- Red beans – 1 can, drained
- Stalks of celery - 2, sliced
- Tomatoes - 1 cup, diced
- Carrots - 2, diced
- White beans - 1 can, drained
- Chicken stock - 4 cups
- Water - 4 cups
- Tomato paste - 1 tbsp.
- Pasta - ½ cup
- Salt and pepper - to taste
- Lemon juice - 2 tbsp.

Directions:
1. Add olive oil to a pot and heat.
2. Add in the sausages and cook for 5 minutes to cook through. Add vegetables and cook for 10 minutes.
3. Pour in all liquid INGREDIENTS: and pasta and add salt and pepper to taste.
4. Set heat to low and cook for an additional 25 minutes. Serve soup warm or chilled.

Cozy Cod Soup

Servings 8
Preparation time: 1 hour
INGREDIENTS:
- Olive oil - 2 tbsp.
- Carrot - 1, sliced
- Red bell pepper - 1, cored and diced
- Shallots - 2, chopped
- Celery – 1 stalk, sliced
- Garlic cloves - 2, chopped
- Marjoram - ½ tsp.
- Marjoram - ½ tsp.
- Potatoes - 1 ½ lbs., peeled and cubed
- Tomatoes - 1 cup, diced
- Cod fillets - 4, cubed

- Bay leaf - 1 leaf
- Thyme - 1 sprig
- Water - 6 cups
- Lemon juice - 2 tbsp.
- Chicken stock - 2 cups
- Salt and pepper - to taste

Directions:
1. Heat olive oil in a pot and add garlic, shallots, bell pepper, celery, and carrot.
2. After cooking for 5 minutes you will add in bay leaf, marjoram, stock, tomatoes, water, potatoes, thyme, and marjoram.
3. Add in salt and pepper to suit your taste and lower heat, cooking an additional 20 minutes.
4. Place cod in the pot, add lemon juice and cook for 5 more minutes. Serve right away.

Chicken Sausage Soup

Servings 10
Preparation time: 1 hour
INGREDIENTS:
- Chicken sausage 6, sliced
- Olive oil - 3 tbsp.
- Red bell peppers – 2, cored and diced
- Shallots - 2, sliced
- Celery stalk - 1, diced
- Tomatoes - 1 can, diced
- Carrots – 2, diced
- Bow tie pasta - 1 cup
- Vegetable stock - 4 cups
- Water - 4 cups
- Dried oregano - 1 tsp.
- Salt and pepper - to taste
- Parsley – 2 tbsp., chopped
- Dried basil - 1 tsp.
- Cilantro - 2 tbsp., chopped

Directions:
1. Heat olive oil in a saucepan or soup pot and then add sausage.
2. Heat sausage for 5 minutes until cooked through and add the celery, bell peppers, shallots, tomatoes and carrots.
3. After 5 minutes, add in water, stock, salt, pepper, oregano, basil and pasta, cooking for an additional 25 minutes.
4. Add cilantro and parsley. Soup is done and ready to serve.

White Bean Vegetable Soup

Servings 6
Preparation time: 40 minutes
INGREDIENTS:
- Garlic cloves - 2, chopped
- Carrots - 2, diced
- Olive oil - 2 tbsp.
- Shallots - 2, sliced
- Celery - 2 stalks, sliced
- Chicken stock - 4 cups

- Water - 2 cups
- Rosemary - 1 sprig
- White beans - 2 cans, drained
- Salt and pepper - to taste

Directions:
1. Pour olive oil in a pot and heat.
2. Then add in garlic and shallots, cooking for approximately 5 minutes.
3. Mix in water, stock, rosemary, carrots, beans and celery and season with salt and pepper to suit your taste.
4. Cook an additional 15 minutes. Serve up soup while fresh.

Zucchini Cream Soup

Servings 6
Preparation time: 40 minutes
INGREDIENTS:
- Grated Parmesan – to top soup
- Celery – 1 stalk, sliced
- Olive oil - 2 tbsp.
- Shallot - 1, chopped
- Zucchini - 3, sliced
- Garlic cloves - 2, chopped
- Vegetable stock - 2 cups
- Rosemary - 1 sprig
- Water - 1 cup
- Salt and pepper - to taste
- Heavy cream - ½ cup

Directions:
1. After hearing oil in a pot, mix in shallot, celery and garlic and cook for 5 minutes.
2. Pour in water, stock, rosemary and zucchini.
3. Cook an additional 15 minutes, adding salt and pepper to suit your taste. Remove soup from stove and spoon out the rosemary sprig.
4. Add heavy cream and mix well.
5. Using an immersion blender, puree the soup. Pour into serving bowls and top with cheese, if desired.
6. Soup is ready to eat and is best when hot.

Lemony Chicken and Rice Soup

Servings 8
Preparation time: 1 hour
INGREDIENTS:
- Whole chicken - 1, cut into smaller pieces
- Rosemary - 1 sprig
- Oregano - 1 sprig
- Olive oil - 3 tbsp.
- Thyme - 1 sprig
- Chicken stock - 2 cups
- Lemon juice - 2 tbsp.
- Salt and pepper - to taste
- Water - 6 cups
- Long grain rice - ¼ cup

Directions:
1. Cook chicken in oil that has been heated in a pot, making sure the chicken is browned and cooked through.
2. Add all of the rest of the **INGREDIENTS:**, including salt and pepper to suit your taste.
3. Simmer soup for 40 minutes on low heat.
4. Dish into serving bowls and eat while hot.

Appetizing Lentil Soup (Faki)

Servings: 4
Preparation time: 10 minutes
Cooking time: 20 minutes
INGREDIENTS:
- (14-ounce) can lentils drained
- teaspoon sea salted.
- cup red vinegar.
- bay leaves.
- carrots chopped.
- celery stalks chopped.
- chopped onion
- tablespoons olive oil.
- cans unsalted vegetable soup
- Pinch red pepper flakes

Directions:
1. Put the pot over high heat heat the olive oil until it simmers.
2. Mix the onion carrot and garlic and Cook for 5 to 15 minutes till the vegetables are soft.
3. Add celery and

Directions: for 20 seconds
1. Stir in lentils bay leaves soup sea salt pepper and red pepper flakes.
2. Put any excess water and set the faro aside.
3. Bring it to a simmer. low the heat and simmer for 12 minutes.
4. Remove and discard cove leaves. Stir in the vinegar and serve.

Chicken soup

Servings: 8
Preparation time: 10 minutes
Cooking time: 20 minutes
INGREDIENTS:
- (14-ounce) crushed tomatoes undrained
- fennel bulb, chopped onion.
- tablespoon dried Italian seasoning
- pinch salt.
- 1/2 pinch black pepper.
- 13 ounces boneless skinless sliced chicken breast.
- carrots chopped
- tablespoons olive oil.
- chopped zucchini.
- minced garlic cloves.
- cups unsalted chicken broth

Directions:
1. Put large bowl over high heat until the olive oil begin to simmer.

2. Then add chicken and cooki for about 6 minutes.
3. Remove the chicken from bowl with the help of spoon and put it aside. Add carrots onion red bell pepper and fennel to the oil remaining in the pot.
4. **Directions:** for about 5 minutes stirring occasionally. Add garlic and
5. **Directions:** for 30 seconds stirring constantly. Stir in the broth tomatoes zucchini. Italian seasoning sea salt and pepper.
6. Bring to a boil stirring occasionally. Reduce the heat and simmer for about 5 minutes more. Return the chicken to the pot.
7. **Directions:** for 1 minute more until the chicken heats through. Serve immediately.

Tasty Zucchini and Meatball Soup

Servings: 6
Preparation time: 20 minutes
Cooking time: 25 minutes
INGREDIENTS:

- 1 (14-ounce) can chopped tomatoes drained
- 1 red onion.
- 1 pinch Italian seasoning.
- 1 pinch garlic powder
- 1 pinch sea salt. pinch black pepper.
- 1/4 cup chopped basil leaves.
- 12 ounces ground turkey
- 1yellow onion grated and squeezed of excess water
- tablespoons extra-virgin olive oil
- medium zucchini chopped or spiralized garlic cloves.
- cups unsalted chicken broth

Directions:
1. In a medium bowl mix together the turkey yellow onion. Italian seasoning garlic powder.
2. On plate to combination into 3/4-inch balls and put aside. Put the bowl over a medium heat and begin to heat olive oil till it simmers.
3. Add red onion and cook for about 5 minutes stirring occasionally until soft. Now add garlic and cook for 20 seconds stirring constantly.
4. Stir in the broth. Bring to a boil.
5. Add the meatballs and return to a boil. Reduce the heat to medium-low. Simmer for about 15 minutes stirring occasionally until the meatballs are through. Add the zucchini and
6. **Directions:** for about 3 minutes more until soft. Stir in the basil just before serving.

Soup chunky for the Mediterranean

Cooking and preparation: 1 hour
Serves: 8
INGREDIENTS:

- extra virgin olive oil – 2 tbsps
- chopped shallot - 1
- minced garlic cloves - 1
- peeled and cubed eggplants - 1
- cubed zucchini - 1
- cored and diced red bell peppers - 2
- diced tomatoes – 1 can
- drained white beans – 1 can
- water – 8 cups

- thyme sprig - 1
- oregano sprig – 1
- Pepper and salt to taste
- Juiced lemon - 1
- chopped parsley – 2 tbsps

Directions:
1. Stir in the garlic and shallot a heated oil contained in a soup pot.
2. Cook it for about 5 minutes after adding zucchini, the eggplants and bell peppers, and stir in the remaining **INGREDIENTS:** apart from parsley and the lemon juice.
3. Cook it for 25 minutes after seasoning with pepper and salt and cook on low heat.
4. Cook for 5 minutes more after adding the lemon juice.
5. The soup is best enjoyed when served fresh and warm.

Special Orzo Soup

Cooking and preparation: 45 minutes.
Serves: 8
INGREDIENTS:
- Orzo – ¼ cup
- vegetable stock – 2 cups
- lemon juice – 2 tbsps
- cored and diced yellow bell pepper - 1
- extra virgin olive oil – 2 tbsps
- chopped shallots - 2
- baby spinach – 4 cups
- green peas – 1 cup
- cored and diced green bell pepper - 1
- water – 4 cups
- chopped garlic cloves - 2
- Pepper and salt to taste

Directions:
1. In a soup pot, heat the oil and stir in the garlic and shallots.
2. Add other **INGREDIENTS:** after cooking it for 2 minutes and season with pepper and salt.
3. On low heat, cook it for 25 minutes. Best served chilled or warm.

Delicious Meatball Soup for the Spanish

Cooking and preparation: 1 hour
Serves: 8
INGREDIENTS:
- water – 6 cups
- crushed tomatoes – 1 can
- egg - 1
- olive oil – 2 tbsps
- diced celery stalk - 1
- chopped onion – 1
- cored and diced red bell peppers – 2
- vegetable stock – 2 cups
- diced carrots - 2
- pound ground veal - 1
- chopped parsley – 2 tbsps
- chopped garlic cloves - 2

- Pepper and salt to taste

Directions:

1. In a soup pot, heat the oil and stir in the garlic, stock, bell peppers, onions, carrots, water and celery.
2. Bring to a boiling after seasoning with pepper and salt. In a bowl, mix egg, veal and parsley in the meantime.
3. Then boil them in boiling liquid after forming small meatballs.
4. Adjust the taste with pepper and salt after adding the tomatoes. For 20 minutes, cook on heat that is very low.
5. Best served fresh and warm.

Delicious and entertaining Lamb Veggie Soup

Cooking and preparation: 1 ½ hours
Serves: 8
INGREDIENTS:

- water – 6 cups
- cubed pound lamb shoulder – 1 1 2
- lemon juice – 2 tbsps
- cauliflower florets – 2 cups
- olive oil – 2 tbsps
- basil sprig - 1
- chopped shallots – 2
- crushed tomatoes – 1 can
- diced carrots – 2
- thyme sprig - 1
- diced celery stalks – 2
- green peas – ½ cup
- grated ginger – ¼ tsp
- vegetable stock – 4 cups
- oregano sprig - 1
- Pepper and salt to taste

Directions:

1. In a soup pot, heat the oil and stir in the lamb shoulder.
2. Add stock and water after cooking on all sides for 5 minutes.
3. Add the remaining **INGREDIENTS:** after cooking for 40 minutes and season with pepper and salt.
4. Cook it for another 20 minutes and serve the soup when it's still fresh.

Italian Lentil soup

INGREDIENTS:

- 2 tablespoons of sliced parsley
- Tomato paste; 2 tablespoons
- Olive Oil; 2 tablespoons
- 2 sliced cloves
- 1 cup of sliced tomatoes
- 2 celery stalks; chopped
- 2 sliced shallots
- 2 carrots; chopped
- ¼ cup of red wine
- Water; 6 cups

- A basil sprig
- A thyme sprigs
- An oregano sprig
- Green lentils; 1 cup
- 2 cups of vegetable stock
- Pepper and salt to taste

Directions:
1. Get a soup pot and heat your olive oil, then pour in your chopped celery, clove, carrots and shallot, then cook for 5 minutes before adding your vegetable stock, lentils, tomatoes, wine and water.
2. Join in the herbs, then add pepper and salt to taste and then cook for 25 minutes.
3. After 25 minutes, add your sliced parsley in and serve your warm soup.

Roasted Vegetable soup

INGREDIENTS:
- Vegetable stock; 2 cups
- 2 sliced red bell pepper
- 4 tomatoes; diced
- 2 cups of water
- A sprig of rosemary
- Olive oil; 3 tablespoons
- 1 sliced carrot
- 2 red onions; cut in halves
- 4 cloves
- Pepper and salt to taste
- A small butternut; crushed, peeled and diced

Directions:
1. Get a baking tray and add your carrot, cloves, tomatoes, red onions, parsnip, bell pepper, rosemary and crushed butternut.
2. Add pepper and salt to taste then drizzle with oil
3. Now, preheat your oven to 350F, then cook for 25-30 minutes till it turns golden brown.
4. Move your vegetable into a soup pot and add in the stock and some water then cook for another 10 minutes.
5. After 10 minutes, remove the rosemary then grind with an immersion blender.
6. Enjoy your soup when warm.

Mediterranean Bean and Sausage soup

INGREDIENTS:
- Olive oil; 2 tablespoons
- A can of drained black beans
- Juiced tomato; 1 cup
- 4 cups of water
- 1 pound of sliced chicken sausage
- 2 cups of chicken stalk
- 1 chopped celery stalk
- 2 sliced cloves
- 1 can of drained kidney beans
- 1 sliced carrot
- 2 peeled and sliced tomatoes
- A rosemary sprig

- 1 bay leaf
- A sweet onion; diced
- Pepper and salt to taste

Directions:
1. Get a soup pot and heat your olive oil, then pour in your sausage and cook for 5 minutes.
2. Now, add all other **INGREDIENTS:**. Add pepper and salt to taste and cook for 25 minutes.
3. Serve and enjoy when cooled

Red Beet soup

INGREDIENTS:
- Vegetable stock; 4 cups
- Water; 2 cups
- 2 sliced carrots
- Olive oil; 2 tablespoons
- 2 sliced leeks
- 1 sliced parsnip
- Shredded cabbage; 2 cups
- 2 peeled and sliced red beets
- A sprig of rosemary
- 1 sliced celery stalk
- A sprig of thyme
- Diced tomatoes; 1 cup
- 1 bay leaf
- Pepper and salt to taste

Directions:
1. Get a soup pot and heat your olive oil, then add in your sliced celery, leeks, parsnip, carrots, beets and your shredded cabbage and cook for 5 minutes.
2. Now, add the rest of your **INGREDIENTS:** with pepper and salt to taste and cook for 20-25 minutes.
3. Serve and enjoy when cooled.

Seafood Tomato soup

INGREDIENTS:
- Diced tomatoes; 1 can
- 2 diced cod fillet
- ¼ cup of white wine
- Water; 3 cups
- Worcestershire sauce; 1 teaspoon
- 2 cups of vegetable stock
- ½ pound rinsed scallops
- 4 sliced cloves
- 1 sliced celery stalk
- Olive oil; 2 tablespoons
- 1 sliced sweet onion
- Lemon juice; 2 tablespoons
- 1 jelapeno pepper; sliced
- 1 pound of peeled and deveined shrimp
- Pepper and salt to taste

Directions:

1. Get a soup pot and heat your olive oil, then pour in your jelapeno, clove, celery then cook for 5 minutes.
2. Add your stock, diced tomatoes, wine and water, then add pepper and salt to taste and cook for 15 minutes.
3. Now, add the remaining INGREDIENTS: and cook for another 10 minutes.
4. Serve and enjoy your soup

Italian meatball Soup

INGREDIENTS:

- Ground chicken; 1 pound
- Chicken stock; 4 cups
- Chopped parsley; 2 tablespoons
- 1 juiced lemon
- 1 sliced shallot
- Water; 4 cups
- ½ teaspoon of dried oregano
- White rice; 2 tablespoons
- Tomato juice; 1 cup
- 1 sliced carrot
- 2 cored and sliced red bell pepper
- 2 sliced tomatoes
- 1 sliced celery stalk
- Dried basil; 1 teaspoon
- Pepper and salt to taste

Directions:

1. Get a soup pot and add your sliced tomatoes, bell pepper, celery, stock, basil, carrot, oregano, tomato juice, shallot and water together, then add pepper and salt to taste and cook for 10 minutes.
2. Create meatballs by combining your white rice, chicken and parsley together.
3. Create small meatballs and drop them in the soup, then cook for another 15 minutes.
4. Add lemon juice. Serve and enjoy.

Veal Shank Barley soup

INGREDIENTS:

- ½ cup of rinsed barley pearls
- 1 sliced sweet onion
- 2 sliced carrots
- 2 peeled and sliced tomatoes
- Vegetable stock; 4 cups
- Olive Oil; 3 tablespoons
- 2 cored and sliced red bell pepper
- Chopped parsley for serving
- 4 sliced veal shank
- 2 chopped celery stalk
- 1 sliced parsnip
- Water; 4 cups
- Pepper and salt to taste

Directions:

1. Get a soup pot and heat your olive oil, then pour in your sliced veal shank and cook for 10 minutes, then add in your stock with water and cook for 10 minutes.
2. Now, add your the rest of your INGREDIENTS: except the chopped parsley.
3. Cook for another 30 minutes on low heat then add pepper and salt to taste.
4. Serve and enjoy your soup topped with parsley.

Tuscan Cabbage soup

INGREDIENTS:

- 1 shredded cabbage
- 2 diced sweet onion
- A sprig of oregano
- Water; 2 cups
- Olive oil; 2 tablespoons
- 1 sliced celery stalk
- 1 sprig of thyme
- 1 sprig of basil
- Vegetable stock; 2 cups
- 2 grated carrot
- 1 juiced lemon
- Diced tomatoes; 1 can
- Pepper and salt to taste

Directions:

1. Get a soup pot and heat your olive oil, then add in your celery, carrots and onions then cook for 5 minutes before adding the rest of your INGREDIENTS:.
2. Add pepper and salt to taste then cook for 25 minutes on low heat.
3. Serve and enjoy

Chickpea Soup with yoghurt

Cooking and preparation: 45 minutes.
Serves: 4
INGREDIENTS:

- Water – 2 cups
- Chopped shallot – 1
- Greek yogurt – ½ cup
- Diced celery stalk – 1
- Crushed tomatoes – 1 can
- Drained chickpeas – 1 can
- Vegetable stock – 2 cups
- Pepper and salt to taste
- Olive oil – 2 tbsps

Directions:

1. Stir in a soup pot shallot, celery and heated oil.
2. Allow it to soften by cooking it for 2 minutes.
3. Then add other **INGREDIENTS:** like stock, chickpeas, water, pepper, tomatoes and salt. Cook for 15 minutes on low heat.
4. Stir the soup in the yogurt after removing it from heat.
5. Then use an immersion blender to puree the soup so that it can be smooth and creamy. It's best served fresh

Pasta and pizza

Olive Oil Pizza Dough

ENERGY VALUE PER PORTION
CALORIE CONTENT392KCAL
SQUIRRELS9.8GRAM
FATS6.3GRAM
CARBOHYDRATES75,4GRAM
INGREDIENTS

- Water ⅔ cup
- Wheat flour 2 cups
- Dry yeast 1 teaspoon
- Salt 1 teaspoon
- 1 tablespoonolive oil

COOKING INSTRUCTION 30 MINUTES

1. Pour the yeast with warm water. Stir the mixture properly so that there are no lumps.
2. Pour 2 cups flour and salt into a large bowl. Add yeast and knead the dough.
3. Put the dough out of the bowl on a dry, floured surface, and continue to knead, adding flour if necessary, until the dough is soft and elastic (about 10 minutes).
4. Lightly grease a large bowl with olive oil. Put the dough in a bowl, turning it so that the entire surface is smeared with oil.
5. Cover with a film and place in a warm, without drafts, place for 1.5 hours (until the dough increases about 2 times).
6. Flatten the dough with your fists. Divide into 2 parts and roll into balls.

Crispy Pizza Dough

CENERGY VALUE PER PORTION
CALORIE CONTEN T495 KCAL
SQUIRRELS 13.8 GRAM
FATS 15.4 GRAM
CARBOHYDRATES 76.3 GRAM
INGREDIENTS

- Wheat flour 2 cups
- 2 tablespoonsolive oil
- ½ cupmilk
- Chicken egg 2 pieces
- Saltpinch

COOKING INSTRUCTION 15 MINUTES

1. Heat milk, add eggs and butter, stir.
2. Constantly mixing, pour the milk mixture into the flour, add salt
3. Knead the dough for about 10 minutes to make it elastic.

Thin crispy pizza dough

ENERGY VALUE PER PORTION
CALORIE CONTENT221KCAL
SQUIRRELS6.2GRAM
FATS0.8GRAM
CARBOHYDRATES48GRAM

INGREDIENTS

- Wheat flour 250 g
- Cane sugar 0.3 teaspoon
- Dry yeast 4 g
- 0.4 teaspoonsalt
- Water 125 ml

COOKING INSTRUCTION 1 HOUR 30 MINUTES

1. Prepare the dough. To do this, mix yeast, sugar and 2 tablespoons of warm water in a bowl. Then add 2 tablespoons of flour, mix well again, cover with a towel and put in a warm place for 30 minutes. Watch the dough, it happens that it is ready in 10 minutes!

2. Pour flour into a bowl, make a depression in the middle. Put the dough in the recess, salt, add about 125 ml of warm water. Knead for about 10-15 minutes until the dough is soft, smooth and elastic. It should not stick to your hands, so you may need to add a little flour or water.

3. Cover the dough with a towel and put in a warm place for 1 hour. It should increase in volume by about half.

4. Making a crunch! Heat the oven to 200 degrees, grease the pizza dish with olive oil, roll it out with a diameter of about 28 cm, put it in the mold, form the sides (or not), grease with tomato sauce and put in the oven for about 5 minutes.

5. Then remove, distribute the rest of the filling and bake for another 20 minutes. Due to the fact that the dough is slightly baked at the beginning, it will become crispy, but at the same time it will not burn!

Yeast Pizza Dough

ENERGY VALUE PER PORTION
CALORIE CONTENT 394 KCAL
SQUIRRELS 9.8 GRAM
FATS 5.8 GRAM
CARBOHYDRATES 76.9 GRAM
INGREDIENTS

- Wheat flour 2 cups
- Vegetable oil 1 tablespoon
- Fresh yeast 20 g
- Sugar 1 teaspoon
- Salt 1 teaspoon

COOKING INSTRUCTION 20 MINUTES

1. In one glass of warm water, dilute 20 grams of yeast (or 1/3 sachet of dry yeast). Leave to stand for 10 minutes.

2. Add 1 tablespoon of vegetable oil, pour all this into 2 cups flour, add salt and sugar.

3. Knead the dough well.

Fresh Sour Cream Pizza Dough

ENERGY VALUE PER PORTION
CALORIE CONTENT 333 KCAL
SQUIRRELS 7.9 GRAM
FATS 10.8 GRAM
CARBOHYDRATES 51.9 GRAM
INGREDIENTS

- Wheat flour 200 g
- Sour cream 200 g

COOKING INSTRUCTION 15 MINUTES

1. Knead the dough from flour and sour cream, divide into 3 equal parts, roll each part into a thin circle.

2. Put on a baking sheet, put the filling.

Fast, yeast-free pizza dough
ENERGY VALUE PER PORTION
CALORIE CONTENT 468 KCAL
SQUIRRELS 14 GRAM
FATS 15.6 GRAM
CARBOHYDRATES 68.7 GRAM
INGREDIENTS

- Wheat flour 350 g
- Kefir 250 ml
- Chicken egg 2 pieces
- Olive oil 40 ml
- ¼ teaspoonsalt
- ¼ teaspoonsoda

COOKING INSTRUCTION 35 MINUTES

1. Beat eggs with salt in a small bowl.
2. Pour kefir into a large bowl.
3. Add to the kefir soda quenched with vinegar.
4. Pour beaten eggs to kefir, mix well the mixture.
5. Add the flour, I prefer to add it in parts to feel the consistency of the dough. In principle, you can use a blender to prepare the dough, but I prefer to knead this particular dough with my hands.
6. Add olive oil to the dough.
7. Stir the dough. It should be consistency like thick sour cream - liquid, but at the same time it should turn out magnificent - as a result of the reaction of kefir and soda.
8. Lubricate the baking sheet with vegetable oil and pour the quick pizza dough on kefir and put the baking sheet in the oven about 200 degrees. When the dough is browned, you can spread the filling and bake until cooked.

Thin pizza dough with honey

ENERGY VALUE PER PORTION
CALORIE CONTENT 386 KCAL
SQUIRRELS 10.2 GRAM
FATS 4.6 GRAM
CARBOHYDRATES 77.1 GRAM
INGREDIENTS

- Wheat flour 3 cups
- Water 1 cup
- Dry yeast 12 g
- Honey 1.5 teaspoons
- Salt 1 teaspoon
- 1 tablespoonolive oil

COOKING INSTRUCTION 30 MINUTES + 30 MINUTES

1. Heat the water to 60 degrees. Combine half a glass of warm water with yeast (12 grams - 1 sachet) and honey.
2. Separately mix flour, salt, oil.
3. Add the honey-yeast mixture and the remaining water. Knead for at least 5 minutes (the dough should not stick to your hands).
4. Allow the dough to rise in a warm place for 30 minutes (cover with a damp towel so that the dough is not weathered).
5. Knead the dough again for 2 minutes, roll into a circle about 30 cm and put on a baking sheet, pre-oiled. The filling is your choice.

Pasta (pizza dough)

ENERGY VALUE PER PORTION
CALORIE CONTENT562KCAL
SQUIRRELS12,4GRAM
FATS14.1GRAM
CARBOHYDRATES98.1GRAM
INGREDIENTS

- Wheat flour 500 g
- Salt 10 g
- Sugar 15 g
- Water 300 ml
- Olive oil 50 ml
- Dry yeast 7 g

COOKING INSTRUCTION 1 HOUR 40 MINUTES

1. Mix the dry **INGREDIENTS:** flour, salt and sugar.
2. In another bowl, mix water (room temperature), yeast and oil.
3. Combine everything and knead the dough.
4. Leave the dough for an hour, cover with a towel.
5. Distribute on a baking sheet, form the base of the pizza.
6. Lubricate with tomato paste, sprinkle with grated mozzarella and fill the pizza as desired (very tasty with mushrooms and prosciutto, or with tuna and olives), garnish with basil leaves.
7. Bake at 250 degrees for approximately 20–25 minutes.

Pizza dough without yeast in milk

ENERGY VALUE PER PORTION
CALORIE CONTENT 490 KCAL
SQUIRRELS 14 GRAM
FATS 14.6 GRAM
CARBOHYDRATES 76.6 GRAM
INGREDIENTS

- Wheat flour 2 cups
- Milk 125 ml
- Salt 1 teaspoon
- Chicken egg 2 pieces
- Sunflower oil 2 tablespoons

COOKING INSTRUCTION 1 HOUR + 20 MINUTES

1. Making pizza dough without yeast in milk is quite simple. The recipe is designed to prepare a dough, which is enough for two, but only large, baking sheets.
2. Combine flour and salt in one bowl. And in the second butter, milk and eggs, mix well and combine the contents of two bowls in one large container.
3. Wait a few minutes for the whole liquid consistency to soak in the flour, and start mixing the dough. It will take about 15 minutes. Dough, in finished form, should be elastic, soft and smooth.
4. Then you need to take a kitchen towel, of course clean, and soak it in water. As a result, it should be moist, but not wet. Excess fluid must be squeezed out. Wrap the dough in a towel, leave to lie down for 20 minutes.
5. After waiting for the set time, remove the dough and, sprinkling flour on the countertop, roll out, but only very thinly. Place it on a baking sheet and lay out the filling prepared according to your taste preferences. As a result, the finished dough will have an effect that is easy, of course, of puff pastry and has a crispy taste.

Puff pastry pizza

ENERGY VALUE PER PORTION
CALORIE CONTENT 746 KCAL
SQUIRRELS 22.8 GRAM
FATS 47.1 GRAM
CARBOHYDRATES 58.3 GRAM
INGREDIENTS

- Puff pastry 500 g
- Sausages 200 g
- Hard cheese 150 g
- Tomatoes 4 pieces
- Dill 1 bunch
- Mayonnaiseto taste
- Tomato pasteto taste
- Champagne Vinegar 150 ml

COOKING INSTRUCTION 30 MINUTES

1. Thaw the dough, roll out, distribute on a baking sheet greased with vegetable oil, make small sides.
2. Sausages cut into rings. Cut the tomatoes into slices. Grate the cheese. Fry the champignons in a pan, add chopped herbs, mix.
3. Grease the dough with tomato paste, put sausages, then tomatoes, grease with mayonnaise, put mushrooms, sprinkle with cheese.
4. Put the pizza in the oven preheated to 180 degrees

Ideal pizza dough (on a large baking sheet)

ENERGY VALUE PER PORTION
CALORIE CONTENT 194 KCAL
SQUIRRELS 5 GRAM
FATS 3.2 GRAM
CARBOHYDRATES 37.1 GRAM
INGREDIENTS

- Wheat flour 375 g
- Salt 1.5 teaspoons
- Dry yeast 1,799 teaspoons
- Sugar 1 teaspoon
- Water 200 ml
- 1 tablespoonolive oil
- Dried Basil 1.5 teaspoons

COOKING INSTRUCTION 1 HOUR

1. We cultivate yeast in warm water. There you can add a spoonful of sugar, so the yeast will begin to work faster. Leave them for 10 minutes.
2. Sift the flour through a sieve (leave 50 g for the future) in a deep bowl. Add salt, basil, mix.
3. Pour water with yeast into the cavity in the flour and mix thoroughly with a fork.
4. Somewhere in the middle of the process, when the dough becomes less than one whole, add olive oil (you can also sunflower).
5. When the dough is ready (it becomes smooth and elastic), cover with a damp towel and put in heat (you can use the battery) for 30 minutes.
6. Now just lay it on a flour dusted surface and roll out the future pizza to a thickness of 2-3 mm.
7. The main rule of pizza is the maximum possible temperature, minimum time. Therefore, feel free to set the highest temperature that is available in your oven.

Vegetable oil pizza dough

ENERGY VALUE PER PORTION
CALORIE CONTENT 222 KCAL
SQUIRRELS 5.8 GRAM
FATS 5.2 GRAM
CARBOHYDRATES 38.5 GRAM
INGREDIENTS

- Wheat flour 1 cup
- Water 1 cup
- Saltto taste
- Vegetable oil 1 tablespoon
- Dry yeast 10 g

COOKING INSTRUCTION 1 HOUR

1. We mix water and yeast, leave for 40 minutes so that they disperse. You can add a tablespoon of sugar.
2. Then pour in the oil, add the flour (here already at the request and degree of tightness of the dough - it should be quite tight, but not too much).
3. Knead well and put in a warm place to increase the volume by 2 times.

Pizza dough on yogurt

ENERGY VALUE PER PORTION
CALORIE CONTENT 336 KCAL
SQUIRRELS 7.3 GRAM
FATS thirteen GRAM
CARBOHYDRATES 48 GRAM
INGREDIENTS

- Natural yogurt 250 g
- Vegetable oil 5 tablespoons
- ½ teaspoonsalt
- Wheat flour 2.5 cups
- Baking powder 1 teaspoon

COOKING INSTRUCTION 30 MINUTES

1. Mix flour, baking powder and salt;
2. Add yogurt and butter, mix everything thoroughly;
3. Preheat the oven to 190 ° C;
4. Lubricate the pan with oil;
5. Roll the dough very thinly and transfer to a baking sheet;
6. Put the filling to taste;
7. Bake for 10-15 minutes.

American Pizza Dough Recipe
ENERGY VALUE PER PORTION
CALORIE CONTENT 769 KCAL
SQUIRRELS 24.2 GRAM
FATS 13.7 GRAM
CARBOHYDRATES 138.5 GRAM
INGREDIENTS

- Wheat flour 170 g
- Chicken egg 1 piece
- Water 85 ml
- Dry yeast 2 g

- Salt 3 g
- Sugar 10 g
- Sunflower oil 5 ml

COOKING INSTRUCTION 15 MINUTES

1. Combine all dry **INGREDIENTS**.
2. Add water and egg. Mix well.
3. After the dough has become homogeneous, gradually add the butter.
4. Leave the dough for 5 minutes.
5. Done! Have a nice evening!

Cuttlefish pasta with carbonara sauce

ENERGY VALUE PER PORTION
CALORIE CONTENT 593 KCAL
SQUIRRELS 22.5 GRAM
FATS 37.5 GRAM
CARBOHYDRATES 40,2 GRAM
INGREDIENTS

- Pasta 200 g
- Smoked bacon 150 g
- Grated Parmesan Cheese 50 g
- Champignons 200 g
- Cream 200 ml
- Egg yolk 1 piece
- Garlic 3 cloves
- Butter 2 tablespoons
- Ground black pepperpinch
- Ground nutmegpinch

COOKING INSTRUCTION 20 MINUTES

1. Boil spaghetti. At this time, fry the garlic and bacon in butter for three minutes.
2. Add the mushroom slices to the bacon, mix and fry for eight to ten minutes. During this time, the spaghetti will cook, drain from them and add to the mushrooms and bacon.
3. The final stage - cream, egg yolk, ground black pepper, ground nutmeg and grated cheese. Beat all this and pour spaghetti, fry for five minutes and serve.

Carbonara pasta with champignons

ENERGY VALUE PER PORTION
CALORIE CONTENT 765 KCAL
SQUIRRELS 32.3 GRAM
FATS 47.8 GRAM
CARBOHYDRATES 50.1 GRAM
INGREDIENTS

- Spaghetti 250 g
- Bacon 200 g
- Cream 20% 200 g
- Parmesan Cheese 100 g
- Egg yolk 4 pieces
- Garlic 5 cloves
- Champignons 150 g
- Olive oil 10 ml
- Saltto taste
- Ground black pepperto taste

COOKING INSTRUCTION 25 MINUTES

1. Prepare the **INGREDIENTS**.
2. Cut the bacon into strips, chop the garlic finely, chop the mushrooms.
3. Fry the garlic in a pan, then the mushrooms and bacon.
4. Grate the parmesan.
5. Put egg yolks in a plate, salt, pepper and beat.
6. Add cream and grated cheese to the yolks, mix.
7. Boil spaghetti to al dente (about a minute less than indicated on the packet).
8. Put the spaghetti in a pan, add the sauce, bacon and mushrooms.

Spaghetti carbonara with red onion

ENERGY VALUE PER PORTION
CALORIE CONTENT 1158 KCAL
SQUIRRELS 46.5 GRAM
FATS 61 GRAM
CARBOHYDRATES 101.8 GRAM
INGREDIENTS

- Spaghetti 250 g
- Butter 20 g
- Garlic 2 cloves
- Red onion 1 head
- Bacon 50 g
- Cream 20% 200 ml
- Grated Parmesan Cheese 50 g
- 4 eggs
- Saltto taste
- Ground black pepperto taste

COOKING INSTRUCTION 20 MINUTES

1. Boil water in a large saucepan and cook the pasta until al dente. Usually for this you need to cook it for a minute less than indicated on the pack.
2. While the pasta is boiling, melt the butter in a pan and fry finely chopped onion, garlic and bacon on it. To softness and to a distinct garlic and fried bacon smell.
3. Remove the pan from the heat and beat four egg yolks with cream and grated Parmesan in a deep bowl. Salt and pepper the mixture, whisk again.
4. In the prepared spaghetti, pour the pieces of bacon fried with onions and garlic. Pour in a mixture of cream, yolks and parmesan, mix. And serve immediately, sprinkled with freshly grated cheese and black pepper

Spaghetti carbonara

ENERGY VALUE PER PORTION
CALORIE CONTENT 715 KCAL
SQUIRRELS 30.5 GRAM
FATS 39,2 GRAM
CARBOHYDRATES 58 GRAM
INGREDIENTS

- Spaghetti 160 g
- Pancetta 120 g
- Hard cheese 50 g
- Egg yolk 2 pieces
- Saltto taste
- Freshly ground black pepperto taste

COOKING INSTRUCTION 30 MINUTES

1. Bring well-salted water to a boil. Cook spaghetti to al dente. Save a little broth from the paste; you may need it. Drain the rest.
2. While preparing the pasta, heat the pan and fry the pancetta on it until golden, remove from heat.
3. In a small bowl, beat the yolks with grated cheese until smooth.
4. Return the pan with the pancetta to a small fire, add about 50 ml of the broth from the pasta, throw the spaghetti there and mix well until the boiling stops. Most of the water should boil.
5. Remove the pan from the heat and add the yolks with cheese and mix quickly until the yolks thicken. If the sauce seems too thick, add a little more paste broth. Pepper and salt to taste, serve.

Chanterelle Pasta

ENERGY VALUE PER PORTION
CALORIE CONTENT 360 KCAL
SQUIRRELS 16.9 GRAM
FATS 16.1 GRAM
CARBOHYDRATES 35.7 GRAM
INGREDIENTS

- Chanterelles 200 g
- Tagliatelle pasta 200 g
- Tomato Sauce 200 g
- Garlic 2 cloves
- Olive oil 20 ml
- Dry white wine 30 ml
- Butter 10 g
- Parmesan Cheese 50 g
- Saltto taste
- Ground black pepperto taste

COOKING INSTRUCTION 15 MINUTES

1. Heat olive oil in a pan with a thick bottom, add a couple of whole cloves of garlic, add chanterelles (pre-washed and well-dried).
2. Fry the chanterelles 5-7 minutes until golden brown, pour in white wine, evaporate.
3. Then pour the tomato sauce and simmer for about 5 minutes. At the end, add butter, salt and pepper.
4. Add the paste cooked al-dente to the sauce and mix. Serve garnished with sliced parmesan and parsley.

Pasta "Verochka"

ENERGY VALUE PER PORTION
CALORIE CONTENT 686 KCAL
SQUIRRELS 24.2 GRAM
FATS 31.1 GRAM
CARBOHYDRATES 74,2 GRAM
INGREDIENTS

- Spaghetti 300 g
- Cream 33% 200 ml
- Lightly salted trout 100 g
- Grated Parmesan Cheese 50 g
- Dried oreganoto taste
- Dried basilto taste

COOKING INSTRUCTION 13 MINUTES

1. Boil spaghetti - or other suitable pasta - until cooked, following the time indicated on the package. You do not need to salt water - the salt will give the fish.
2. Meanwhile, finely chop the red fish - not necessarily trout, any. And its quantity may be different - if only the fish had no more pasta.
3. Heat the cream in a pan (it is better to take fatter) and add fish to them. Keep on fire, stirring constantly and, most importantly, not boiling. When the fish loses color, you can remove the pan from the heat.
4. Throw the prepared pasta into a colander and add to the sauce. Or add the sauce to the paste - as anyone is more familiar and convenient. Add oregano and basil, mix.
5. Sprinkle the paste spread on the plates with grated Parmesan.

Pasta e patate

ENERGY VALUE PER PORTION
CALORIE CONTENT 615 KCAL
SQUIRRELS 23,2 GRAM
FATS 29.9 GRAM
CARBOHYDRATES 63.1 GRAM
INGREDIENTS

- Bacon 140 g
- Onions 80 g
- Spaghetti 240 g
- Potato400 g
- Parmesan Cheese 80 g
- Olive oil 30 ml
- Freshly ground black pepperto taste
- Saltto taste

COOKING INSTRUCTION 30 MINUTES

1. Fry the bacon in a dry skillet. Add olive oil and fry finely chopped onions, not until golden brown.
2. Add chopped potatoes to the onion, fry and add water to the onion. Cook until al dente, 5-10 minutes.
3. Break the spaghetti, toss it to the potatoes, add water, continue cooking until the spaghetti is ready. Pour a little water over the entire cooking process so that a little liquid is left in the finale, sufficient to make a sauce.
4. In the finale add grated parmesan, olive oil, freshly ground black pepper, mix well

Pasta with Fresh Tomatoes

ENERGY VALUE PER PORTION
CALORIE CONTENT 1265 KCAL
SQUIRRELS 45.4 GRAM
FATS 56.2 GRAM
CARBOHYDRATES 136.3 GRAM
INGREDIENTS

- Tagliatelle pasta 200 g
- Tomatoes 1 piece
- 5 black olives
- Garlic 2 cloves
- Olive oil 50 ml

COOKING INSTRUCTION 20 MINUTES

1. Boil the paste in salted boiling water.
2. Simultaneously in 1 tablespoon of olive oil, lightly fry the garlic and sliced olives.

3. Dice the fresh tomatoes and add to the garlic and olives. Cooking tomatoes is not necessary, they should only warm up.
4. Slightly salt and pepper the sauce.
5. Drain the water and combine the pasta with the sauce.
6. Put the pasta in a plate and lightly pour olive oil.

Spaghetti carbonara with chicken

ENERGY VALUE PER PORTION
CALORIE CONTENT 624 KCAL
SQUIRRELS 30.9 GRAM
FATS 29.1 GRAM
CARBOHYDRATES 56.6 GRAM
INGREDIENTS
- Durum wheat spaghetti 300 g
- Cream 100 ml
- Garlic 2 cloves
- Chicken egg 3 pieces
- Basilto taste
- Sesame seeds 15 g
- Saltto taste
- Olive oil 3 tablespoons
- Parmesan Cheese 50 g
- Chicken fillet 200 g

COOKING INSTRUCTION 25 MINUTES
1. Finely chop the chicken fillet and fry in olive oil until tender.
2. Peel the garlic, chop finely and add to the chicken. Fry it all together for 1-2 minutes. Then add cream, salt to taste. Stew on low heat so that the cream does not curl.
3. Add a spoonful of olive oil to boiling water, salt to taste to taste. Cooking spaghetti to al dente.
4. Cooking the sauce. To do this, beat the eggs, then add basil, salt, sesame and grated parmesan.
5. Once the spaghetti is ready, we discard them in a colander, then - in a pan with chicken and garlic, pour everything in the resulting sauce and simmer for another 2-3 minutes over low heat.

Carbonara with fettuccine

ENERGY VALUE PER PORTION
CALORIE CONTENT 916 KCAL
SQUIRRELS 40.9 GRAM
FATS 41,4 GRAM
CARBOHYDRATES 88.1 GRAM
INGREDIENTS
- Fettuccine Pasta 500 g
- Bacon 8 slices
- 4 eggs
- Grated Parmesan Cheese 50 g
- Cream 315 ml

COOKING INSTRUCTION 30 MINUTES
1. Cut the bacon into thin strips and fry in a pan over medium heat until crisp. Lay on a paper towel.
2. Put the pasta in a pot of boiling salted water and cook until cooked. Drain and return to pan.
3. While the pasta is boiling, beat the eggs with cream and parmesan until smooth. Add the bacon and mix well. Pour the sauce into a hot paste and mix well.
4. Return to a frying pan to a very small fire and simmer a little less than 1 minute until the sauce thickens slightly.

Fast Spaghetti Carbonara

ENERGY VALUE PER PORTION
CALORIE CONTENT 841 KCAL
SQUIRRELS 34 GRAM
FATS 49.4 GRAM
CARBOHYDRATES 59.2 GRAM
INGREDIENTS

- Spaghetti 80 g
- Bacon 40 g
- Cream 35% 50 ml
- Chicken egg 1 piece
- Dry white wine 20 ml
- Grana padano cheese 23 g

COOKING INSTRUCTION 15 MINUTES
1. We put spaghetti in boiling water, cook for 12 minutes, put it on a sieve.
2. At the chicken egg, we separate the yolk from the protein, mix the yolks with animal cream, grana padano cheese, and pepper.
3. Cut the bacon with a large plate into large plates, fry in butter, add dry white wine and olive oil.
4. Into the fried bacon with wine and oil we introduce ready-made spaghetti, add the mass with egg and cream, mix quickly

Pasta with garlic and Hoat Pepper

SERVES 4
INGREDIENTS:

- 400g Spaghetti
- 8 tablespoons Extra virgin olive oil
- 4 cloves garlic, chopped
- 1 Chili pepper
- Coarse salt

Directions:
1. Put the water to boil, when it comes to a boil add salt and dip the spaghetti.
2. Meanwhile, in a saucepan heat the oil with the garlic deprived of the inner and chopped germ and the chopped peppers. Be careful: the flame should be sweet and the garlic should not darken.
3. Halfway through cooking, remove the spaghetti and continue cooking in the pan with the oil and garlic, adding the cooking water as if it were a risotto.
4. When cooked, serve the spaghetti.

Each serving contains: Calories 201Kcal, Total Fat 4.3g, Protein 5.8g, Carbohydrate 20.1g, Cholesterol 0mg

Stuffed Pasta Shells

SERVES 4
INGREDIENTS:

- 5 Cups Marinara Sauce
- 15 Ounces Ricotta Cheese
- 1 ½ Cups Mozzarella Cheese, Grated
- ¾ Cup Parmesan Cheese, Grated
- 2 Tablespoons Parsley, Fresh & Chopped
- ¼ Cup Basil Leaves, Fresh & Chopped

- 8 Ounces Spinach, Fresh & Chopped
- ½ Teaspoon Thyme
- Sea Salt & Black Pepper to Taste
- 1 lb. Ground Beef
- 1 Cup Onions, Chopped
- 4 Cloves Garlic, Diced
- 2 Tablespoons Olive Oil, Divided
- 12 Ounces Jumbo Pasta Shells

Directions:

1. Start by cooking your pasta shells by following your package instructions. Once they're cooked, then set them to the side.
2. Press sauté and then add in half of your olive oil. Cook your garlic and onions, which should take about four minutes. Your onions should be tender, and your garlic should be fragrant.
3. Add your ground beef in, seasoning it with thyme, salt, and pepper, cooking for another four minutes.
4. Add in your basil, parsley, spinach and marinara sauce.
5. Cover your pot, and cook for five minutes on low pressure.
6. Use a quick release, and top with cheeses.
7. Press sauté again, making sure that it stays warm until your cheese melts.
8. Take a tablespoon of the mixture, stuffing it into your pasta shells.
9. Top with your remaining sauce before serving warm.

Each serving contains: Calories: 710Kcal, Protein: 45.2 g, Total Fat: 23.1 g, Carbs: 70 g, Cholesterol: 110 g

Homemade pasta bolognese

NERGY VALUE PER PORTION
CALORIE CONTENT 1091 KCAL
SQUIRRELS 52.7 GRAM
FATS 54.7 GRAM
CARBOHYDRATES 92.8 GRAM
INGREDIENTS

- Minced meat 500 g
- Pasta 350 g
- Sweet red onion1 piece
- Garlic 2 cloves
- Vegetable oil 1 tablespoon
- Tomato paste 3 tablespoons
- Grated Parmesan Cheese 50 g
- Bacon3 pieces

COOKING INSTRUCTION 40 MINUTES

1. Fry finely chopped onions and garlic in a frying pan in vegetable oil until a characteristic smell.
2. Add minced meat and chopped bacon to the pan. Constantly break the lumps with a spatula and mix so that the minced meat is crumbly.
3. When the mince is ready, add tomato paste, grated Parmesan to the pan, mix, reduce heat and leave to simmer.
4. At this time, boil the pasta. I don't salt water, because for me tomato paste and sauce as a whole turn out to be quite salty.
5. When the pasta is ready, discard it in a colander, arrange it on plates, add meat sauce with tomato paste on top of each serving.

Penne Bolognese Pasta

ENERGY VALUE PER PORTION
CALORIE CONTENT 862 KCAL
SQUIRRELS 31.8 GRAM
FATS 43,4 GRAM
CARBOHYDRATES 80.3 GRAM
INGREDIENTS

- Penne pasta 200 g
- Beef 150 g
- Parmesan Cheese 30 g
- Celery Stalk 30 g
- Shallots 26 g
- Carrot 40 g
- Garlic 1 clove
- Thyme 1 g
- Tomatoes in own juice 180 g
- Parsley 3 g
- Oregano 1 g
- Butter 20 g
- Dry white wine 50 ml
- Olive oil 40 ml

COOKING INSTRUCTION 30 MINUTES

6. Pour the penne into boiling salted water and cook for 9 minutes.
7. Roll the beef through a meat grinder.
8. Dice onion, celery, carrots and garlic in a small cube.
9. Fry the chopped vegetables in a heated frying pan in olive oil with minced meat for 4–5 minutes, salt and pepper.
10. Add oregano to the fried minced meat and vegetables, pour 50 ml of wine, add the tomatoes along with the juice and simmer for 10 minutes until the tomatoes are completely softened.
11. Add the boiled penne and butter to the sauce and simmer for 1-2 minutes, stirring continuously.
12. Put in a plate, sprinkle with grated Parmesan and chopped parsley, decorate with a sprig of thyme and serve.

Quick pasta bolognese

ENERGY VALUE PER PORTION
CALORIE CONTENT 710 KCAL
SQUIRRELS 34.2 GRAM
FATS 26.8 GRAM
CARBOHYDRATES 80.3 GRAM
INGREDIENTS

- Ground beef 500 g
- Garlic 2 cloves
- Tomato paste 3 tablespoons
- Tomatoes 400 g
- Beef broth 150 ml
- A mixture of Italian herbs1 teaspoon
- Penne pasta 400 g
- Basil leavesto taste
- Fresh mushroomsto taste

COOKING INSTRUCTION 25 MINUTES

1. Prepare the paste following the instructions on the packaging.
2. Heat the oil in a pan, sauté the minced meat for 5 minutes, then add the mushrooms and fry for another 3 minutes. Add garlic and tomato paste and simmer for 2 minutes. Add tomatoes, broth or wine, dried herbs and spices. Bring to a boil and simmer for 10 minutes.

3. Drain the water from the pasta, mix it with the sauce, sprinkle with basil leaves on top.

Pappardelle bolognese

ENERGY VALUE PER PORTION
CALORIE CONTENT 922 KCAL
SQUIRRELS 45.8 GRAM
FATS 69.1 GRAM
CARBOHYDRATES eleven GRAM
INGREDIENTS

- Olive oil 150 ml
- Ground beef 2 kg
- 2 carrots
- Celery stalk 1 piece
- Fresh rosemary 1 piece
- Red onion 2 heads
- Sage 1 piece
- Garlic 2 cloves
- Dry red wine 750 ml
- Tomato paste 1 tablespoon
- Tomato juice 1 l
- Pecorino Romanoto taste
- Saltto taste
- Ground black pepperto taste

COOKING INSTRUCTION 3 HOURS

1. Heat the oil in a deep saucepan with a wide bottom, add finely chopped vegetables, herbs and whole cloves of garlic and fry at high temperature for five to eight minutes, stirring occasionally.

2. Salt and pepper the meat and put it in a pan with vegetables. Stir meat and vegetables from time to time for ten minutes.

3. Then add the wine, mix the contents of the pan and cook until the wine is almost completely evaporated. Remember to stir minced meat and vegetables from time to time.

4. After the wine has almost disappeared from the pan, add the tomato paste first, mix, simmer for three minutes, and then pour the tomato juice with a liter of water. Bring to a boil, then reduce the heat and simmer for one and a half to two hours, sometimes adding a little more water, if necessary, until the mass turns into a thick sauce. You can at this stage move the saucepan to the oven, preheated to 150 degrees. Ragout cooked in the oven will be more intense in taste.

Traditional spaghetti bolognese

ENERGY VALUE PER PORTION
CALORIE CONTENT 988 KCAL
SQUIRRELS 39,2 GRAM
FATS 36.9 GRAM
CARBOHYDRATES 106.1 GRAM
INGREDIENTS

- 2 tablespoonsolive oil
- Garlic 2 cloves
- Onion 1 head

- Carrot 1 piece
- Celery stalk 1 piece
- Dry red wine 375 ml
- Ground beef 500 g
- Beef broth 500 ml
- Sugar 1 teaspoon
- Canned Tomatoes 850 g
- Chopped parsley 3 tablespoons
- Spaghetti 500 g
- Grated Parmesanto taste

COOKING INSTRUCTION 1 HOUR 50 MINUTES

1. Heat olive oil in a large frying pan and add chopped garlic, onions, carrots and celery. Simmer on low heat for 5 minutes until vegetables are tender.

2. Increase the heat and add the meat. Stir with a wooden spatula, breaking the lumps. Add the broth, wine, tomatoes, sugar and parsley. Bring to a boil, reduce heat and simmer for 1.5 hours, stirring occasionally. Salt and add spices.

3. Before serving, cook the spaghetti, drain and serve with the sauce and parmesan.

Vegetarian Bolognese Sauce
ENERGY VALUE PER PORTION
CALORIE CONTENT 422 KCAL
SQUIRRELS 16,2 GRAM
FATS 8 GRAM
CARBOHYDRATES 74.1 GRAM
INGREDIENTS

- 1 tablespoonolive oil
- Garlic 1 clove
- Red onion 1 head
- Carrot 100 g
- Fresh mushrooms 75 g
- Red bell pepper 1 piece
- Tomato paste 500 g
- Broccoli Cabbage 50 g
- Basil leaves ⅓ cup
- Spaghetti 250 g

COOKING INSTRUCTION 30 MINUTES

1. Peel and chop the onion and garlic, peel the carrots and chop thinly into strips. Pepper seed and cut into small pieces.

2. Heat olive oil in a large frying pan and fry chopped onions and garlic on it until soft (but not brown). Add carrots and cook for five minutes, then add pepper and fry for another 2 minutes. Add chopped mushrooms and tomato paste, then add broccoli and basil. Stir and cook for about five minutes until the vegetables are tender.

3. Lightly cool the sauce, then put in a blender bowl and lightly punch - so that the sauce has a delicate, but not uniform texture. Return the sauce to the pan and keep it hot.

Ravioli

ENERGY VALUE PER PORTION
CALORIE CONTENT 500 KCAL
SQUIRRELS 17 GRAM
FATS 6.4 GRAM
CARBOHYDRATES 93 GRAM

INGREDIENTS

- Saltto taste
- Wheat flour 500 g
- Chicken egg 3 pieces

COOKING INSTRUCTION 30 MINUTES

1. Prepare the pastry dough: Pour half the flour into a bowl and deepen in the middle. Send eggs, some water and a pinch of salt. Manually sweep the dough, adding the remaining flour in small pieces. The dough should be firm and smooth. Roll it into a ball, and then throw this ball several times on a table sprinkled with flour - do not spare your strength. Then roll the dough into a ball and leave for 2 hours.

2. Divide the dough in half and roll into two very thin squares. Lay the small pieces of the filling on one of the squares: they should be placed at least 2.5 cm from each other.

3. Moisten the space between the parts of the filling and the second square of the test with water: with wet hands, preferably with a brush. Cover the filling with the second square, wet side down. Then, with a special pasta knife, cut the square into ravioli. If you don't have such a knife, you can cut the ravioli with a regular sharp knife, but first you need to press the strips of dough, passing between the pieces of the filling, to each other so that the ravioli do not fall apart when you cut them. This can be done with a manual fork or knife, or with your fingers.

4. Bring salt water in a large saucepan to a boil. Send the ravioli in parts, and bring it to a boil again. Then turn down the heat and cook for 20 minutes until they are soft. Drain and rinse under cold water so that the ravioli do not stick together.

5. Now they can be mixed with sauce, baked and serve. Ravioli needs to be cooked in such a way as to serve immediately when ready - otherwise, they will dry out.

Mushroom ravioli

ENERGY VALUE PER PORTION
CALORIE CONTENT 501 KCAL
SQUIRRELS 12.8 GRAM
FATS 21.9 GRAM
CARBOHYDRATES 64,2 GRAM
INGREDIENTS

- Wheat flour1 kg
- Water 1.25 cups
- Chicken egg 2 pieces
- Fresh mushrooms 1 kg
- Chives 1 bunch
- 6 tablespoonsolive oil
- Butter 4 tablespoons
- Cream 30% 2 tablespoons
- Hard cheese 1 tablespoon
- Parsley 60 g
- Saltto taste
- Ground black pepperto taste

COOKING INSTRUCTION 1 HOUR 20 MINUTES

1. Knead the dough. Mix flour and salt. Beat eggs with olive oil and water. Pouring the egg mixture into the flour gradually, knead the elastic, elastic dough. Cover the finished dough with a napkin and leave for 30 minutes.

2. Prepare the filling. Finely chop the mushrooms (you can take chanterelles, porcini mushrooms, mushrooms) and onions, fry them in butter. Add cream (you can sour cream), salt, pepper and simmer for 10 minutes. The filling should be juicy.

3. Roll out the dough into 2 identical thin layers. On one layer of dough, spread 1 teaspoon of the filling at a distance of 3-5 cm from each other. Cover with a second layer, firmly press the layers around the filling with your fingers, then cut them into squares.

4. Cook ravioli in boiling salted water for 5-7 minutes. Remove with a slotted spoon, put on a dish, season with oil, sprinkle with grated cheese and herbs. Separately, you can submit ketchup.

Pumpkin Ravioli

ENERGY VALUE PER PORTION
CALORIE CONTENT 835 KCAL
SQUIRRELS 16.3 GRAM
FATS 42.7 GRAM
CARBOHYDRATES 95.5 GRAM
INGREDIENTS

- Coarse flour 200 g
- 4 tablespoonsolive oil
- Mineral waterto taste
- Pumpkin butternut squash 400 g
- Onion 1.5 heads
- Nutmegpinch
- Turmericon the tip of a knife
- Oranges 1 piece
- Tomatoes 1 piece
- Dill ½ beam

COOKING INSTRUCTION 45 MINUTES

1. Making the dough. Add salt and oil to the flour, gradually dilute with the required amount of water, knead until plastic.

2. Make the filling. Cut half a pumpkin (200 g) finely-finely or grate and squeeze the juice. Salt, add half the head of finely chopped onions, turmeric on the tip of the knife and a pinch of nutmeg.

3. Roll out the dough as thinly as possible. Cut ravioli circles (with a glass, cookie cutters or special), if possible, the smallest.

4. We cook in a double boiler for 10 to 15 minutes or in the traditional way - in boiling water on a stove

5. Making the sauce. Finely chop the onion head and fry until golden. The second half of the pumpkin (200 g) is three on a fine grater and poisoned in a frying pan to the already gilded onion, squeeze the orange juice there and simmer for about 5 minutes. After that add the finely chopped garlic clove and tomato, simmer for another 2-3 minutes. Remove from the stove, cover with finely chopped dill and mix.

Beef Ravioli in Chicken Broth

ENERGY VALUE PER PORTION
CALORIE CONTENT 633 KCAL
SQUIRRELS 33,2 GRAM
FATS 28.7 GRAM
CARBOHYDRATES 54.1 GRAM
INGREDIENTS

- Wheat flour 400 g
- Water 1 tablespoon
- 4 eggs
- Beef 500 g
- Onion 1 head
- Carrot 1 piece
- Dry red wine 250 g

- Celery 1 stalk
- Cloves 5 pieces
- Olive oil 50 ml
- Grated Parmesan Cheese 100 g

COOKING INSTRUCTION 1 HOUR 30 MINUTES

1. Mix the flour with salt, collect with a slide, make a deepening in the center, beat in three eggs, add water and fork, mix them with flour, knead the dough for about fifteen minutes, cover with a film, let it rest for half an hour or an hour.

2. Peel vegetables, finely chop, fry in olive oil, add meat, cut into 5 cm slices, fry, stirring, ten minutes, pour wine, simmer for one hour on low heat, cool, strain, put in a blender, salt, beat. , add the yolk of one egg, parmesan and mix.

3. Roll out the dough in a pasta machine, cut out squares with a side of 4-5 cm, put the filling in the middle, make a triangle and then connect two sharp corners. Serve ten to twelve pieces per serving.

4. Cook in chicken broth for three to four minutes, serve with a small amount of broth, sprinkle with parsley on top.

Ravioli with zucchini, arugula and cream cheese

ENERGY VALUE PER PORTION
CALORIE CONTENT 714 KCAL
SQUIRRELS 22.5 GRAM
FATS 34.9 GRAM
CARBOHYDRATES 79.6 GRAM
INGREDIENTS

- Wheat flour 390 g
- Zucchini 500 g
- Mascarpone cheese 200 g
- Arugula 20 g
- 5 egg yolks
- Chicken egg 1 piece
- Cheese 70 g
- Saltto taste

COOKING INSTRUCTION 1 HOUR 30 MINUTES

1. Pour flour onto a table, add salt, make a depression in the middle and pour whipped yolks. Gently mix the yolks with flour and knead the dough. If it turns out to be too steep, add some room temperature water.

2. Knead the dough for ten minutes until it becomes elastic. Then form a ball from the dough and tightly wrap it with cling film. Put in the refrigerator for at least half an hour.

3. Grate one large zucchini on a coarse grater with the skin, put in a colander, salt and set aside for a while, periodically squeezing the liquid. Grind a handful of arugula. Grate hard cheese.

4. In a bowl, mix with a spoon grated zucchini with arugula, grated hard cheese and mascarpone to a homogeneous, tender, but not liquid minced meat.

5. Remove the dough from the refrigerator and roll it into a layer 1.5–2 mm thick. It's better, of course, to do this with the help of a pasta machine, but if it is not there, either brute masculine strength or a very heavy rolling pin — for example, marble — will help.

6. Mark the cups on the dough with a glass, put in the center of each cup a full teaspoon of the filling. Lubricate the dough around the filling with a beaten egg. Cover on top with another layer of dough and squeeze the dough well, squeezing out all the air around the filling.

7. Cut the mugs out with a glass and seal them well at the edges. Leave the ravioli for about an hour to allow them to dry. Then boil water in a saucepan, slightly salt and put ravioli. Cook for three to four minutes.

8. Put the prepared ravioli with a slotted spoon on heated plates and serve hot by pouring with melted butter or homemade pesto.

Spinach and Tomato Salsa Ravioli

ENERGY VALUE PER PORTION
CALORIE CONTENT 506 KCAL
SQUIRRELS 21.1 GRAM
FATS 21.7 GRAM
CARBOHYDRATES 57.1 GRAM
INGREDIENTS

- Wheat flour 400 g
- Water 1 tablespoon
- 4 eggs
- Spinach 100 g
- Ricotta cheese 300 g
- Grated Parmesan Cheese 50 g
- Nutmeg 1 teaspoon
- Butter 15 g
- Onions ½ heads
- Celery stalk with leaves 1 piece
- Tomatoes 3 pieces
- Carrot 1 piece
- Basil 50 g
- Olive oil 30 ml
- Saltto taste

COOKING INSTRUCTION 1 HOUR

1. Mix the flour with salt, collect in a slide, in the center make a recess, drive in three eggs, add water and mix them with flour with a fork. Knead the dough for about fifteen minutes, then cover it with foil and let it rest for half an hour or an hour.
2. Wash the spinach, fry with one teaspoon of butter for five minutes, chop finely, mix with ricotta, parmesan, nutmeg, add a pinch of salt, beat an egg, mix well and refrigerate.
3. For the sauce, peel the onions, carrots and celery, finely chop, fry for three minutes without oil in a saucepan, add the tomatoes, stew for half an hour, rub through a sieve or grind into porridge in a blender.
4. Roll out the dough in a paste machine, put the filling on one teaspoon on one sheet every 5 cm, cover with a second sheet of dough, press the upper sheet to the lower sheet with your fingers and cut out 5x5 cm squares with a knife.

Homemade Ravioli with Ricotta and Spinach

ENERGY VALUE PER PORTION
CALORIE CONTENT 465 KCAL
SQUIRRELS 22 GRAM
FATS 15.8 GRAM
CARBOHYDRATES 60.3 GRAM
INGREDIENTS

- Wheat flour 300 g
- 4 eggs
- Ricotta cheese 250 g
- Frozen Spinach 100 g
- Ground nutmegpinch
- Grated Parmesanto taste
- Saltto taste
- Ground black pepperto taste

COOKING INSTRUCTION 1 HOUR

1. Pour flour onto a table, make a depression in the middle and pour 3 eggs. Gently mix the eggs with flour. Knead the dough for another eight to ten minutes, until it becomes elastic. Then wrap in foil and leave in the refrigerator for at least half an hour.

2. In a deep bowl, combine ricotta, spinach and 1 egg, add a pinch of nutmeg, salt and pepper to taste. If the spinach is frozen, it should only be thawed, if fresh, blanch for three to four minutes and chop.

3. Roll out the dough into strips 1–1.5 mm thick. It is more convenient to do this with a pasta machine.

4. Observing equal intervals, put the filling on the dough, about 1 teaspoon. Cover on top with another layer of dough and squeeze well, squeezing out all the air around the filling. Trim excess dough with a knife or a special form for ravioli.

5. Boil fresh ravioli in salted boiling water for four to five minutes. Serve sprinkled with grated Parmesan.

Apple Ravioli

ENERGY VALUE PER PORTION
CALORIE CONTENT 372 KCAL
SQUIRRELS 9.9 GRAM
FATS 8.9 GRAM
CARBOHYDRATES 63.8 GRAM
INGREDIENTS

- Wheat flour 400 g
- 4 eggs
- Vegetable oil 2 tablespoons
- Apple 4 pieces
- Bananas 2 pieces
- Lemon 1 piece
- Raisins 60 g
- Ground cinnamonto taste
- Sugarto taste
- Saltto taste

COOKING INSTRUCTION 1 HOUR 30 MINUTES

1. Mix the flour with a pinch of salt and oil, then grind the mixture into crumbs. Separate the yolks from the proteins. Add the yolks to the crumbs and, pouring warm water over a tablespoon, knead the elastic dough. Roll the dough into a ball, keep in the refrigerator for 1 hour.

2. Prepare the filling. Dice apples, combine with sliced bananas, sprinkle with freshly squeezed lemon juice, add seedless raisins, sugar, cinnamon, mix.

3. Roll out the dough into 2 thin layers. Put 2 teaspoons of the filling on one layer with an interval of 6 cm. Grease the distance between the filling with protein, cover with a second layer, press the dough with your fingers around the filling, connecting the layers, and cut into separate ravioli with a dough roller.

4. Dip ravioli in boiling salted water and cook for 8 minutes. When serving, put the finished ravioli on a plate, sprinkle with cinnamon, arrange with lemon balm and cranberry or strawberry jam.

Cheese Ravioli

ENERGY VALUE PER PORTION
CALORIE CONTENT 1186 KCAL
SQUIRRELS 38,4 GRAM
FATS 84.3 GRAM
CARBOHYDRATES 65.3 GRAM
INGREDIENTS

- Coarse flour 400 g
- 8 tablespoonsolive oil

- Mineral waterto taste
- Spinach 300 g
- Leek 1 piece
- Feta Cheese 400 g
- Dried Mushrooms 30 g
- Saltto taste
- Fresh thymeto taste
- Cream Cheese 350 g

COOKING INSTRUCTION 20 MINUTES

1. Pour the flour into a deep bowl, add a pinch of salt and oil. Gradually adding the required amount of water, knead the plastic dough.

2. In a separate bowl, grate the cheese on a coarse grater. Grind spinach and leek, mix in cheese.

3. In a mortar, grind salt, thyme and dried mushrooms. Add to the filling and mix well. Allow to stand for several minutes.

4. On a work surface, thinly roll out the dough and cut it using a mold for making Italian ravioli dumplings of the desired shape. Put a full teaspoon of the filling on each circle of dough.

5. Place ravioli in a double boiler and cook for 15 minutes. Serve on warmed dishes, garnish with a mixture of canned beans, corn, tomato sauce or pesto.

Ricotta with Ricotta and Spinach
ENERGY VALUE PER PORTION
CALORIE CONTENT 1287 KCAL
SQUIRRELS 56.2 GRAM
FATS 48.7 GRAM
CARBOHYDRATES 157 GRAM
INGREDIENTS

- Wheat flour 400 g
- Egg yolk 2 pieces
- Chicken egg 2 pieces
- Salt1 teaspoon
- Spinach 200 g
- Ricotta cheese 300 g
- Butter 20 g
- Water 1 cup
- Parmesan Cheese 50 g

COOKING INSTRUCTION 25 MINUTES

1. Rinse and chop the spinach, mix with ricotta.

2. Lightly beat the eggs in the combine, add salt, flour and yolks and mix in the combine. The resulting dough is divided into two parts and rolled into thin layers.

3. On one layer of dough, spread the filling with balls at a distance of 5 cm from each other. Cover with a second layer. Cut into squares and put in the freezer for 10 minutes.

4. In a pan with a thick bottom, heat the oil, add a glass of broth (or water), salt. Cook ravioli under the lid for 10 minutes. Pepper and sprinkle with parmesan.

Lamb ravioli

ENERGY VALUE PER PORTION
CALORIE CONTENT 1220 KCAL
SQUIRRELS 18.7 GRAM
FATS 108.6 GRAM
CARBOHYDRATES 44.8 GRAM
INGREDIENTS

- Fresh cilantro (coriander) 6 g
- Lamb 200 g

- Lamb broth 770 ml
- Onion 30 g
- Gedza dumplings dough 300 g
- Chicken egg 1 piece
- Cherry Tomatoes 300 g
- Fresh thyme 5 g
- Garlic 5 cloves
- Olive oil 100 ml
- Butter 350 g
- Salt to taste
- Ground black pepper to taste

COOKING INSTRUCTION 40 MINUTES

1. Remove lamb flesh from excess fat and films, pass through a meat grinder with a fine grill. Chop onion into small cubes, chop cilantro, mix with minced meat. Pour 20 ml of broth into the minced meat, salt and pepper to taste, mix everything well.

2. Ready rice dough for gedza divided into circles. Grease a circle of rice dough with a slightly beaten egg, put the minced meat, cover with a second circle, pinch the edges, pushing out excess air. Trim the edges with a curly mold.

3. Fry shallots, chopped into small cubes, in a deep pan in olive oil, along with crushed garlic cloves and thyme leaves. Add the broth and evaporate to about half the volume.

4. Add the cherry tomatoes and butter cut in half. Evaporate to a sauce consistency.

5. While preparing the sauce, boil the ravioli in salted boiling water for about 3-4 minutes until cooked and transfer the finished ravioli to the pan with the sauce so that everything goes together. Bring the dish to taste with salt and pepper, put the ravioli in a plate and pour the sauce. You can decorate with branches of fresh young cilantro.

Ravioli Milan

ENERGY VALUE PER PORTION
CALORIE CONTENT 612 KCAL
SQUIRRELS 27.1 GRAM
FATS 26.2 GRAM
CARBOHYDRATES 68.8 GRAM
INGREDIENTS

- Wheat flour 500 g
- Water 4 tablespoons
- Chicken egg 2 pieces
- Parsley 1 bunch
- Minced pork 400 g
- Dill 1 bunch
- Chervil ½ beam
- Garlic 2 cloves
- Onion 1 head
- Grated Parmesan cheese 2 tablespoons
- Butter 1 tablespoon
- Tomato Sauce 250 g
- 1.5 l meat broth
- Salt to taste
- Ground black pepper to taste
- Nutmeg pinch

COOKING INSTRUCTION 1 HOUR 30 MINUTES

1. Drive eggs into the flour, add warm water, salt, knead the dough, cover with a towel and leave for 20 minutes.

2. Mix the minced meat with finely chopped onions, garlic and herbs, season with salt, pepper, nutmeg and a piece of cheese. Mix everything well and fry in oil, stirring occasionally.

3. Divide the dough in half, roll each half very thinly. Put the filling on one half with a teaspoon with an interval of 2 cm. Moisten the dough with water, cover with the second half. Press the dough around the filling and cut out the squares with a gear knife.

4. Dip ravioli in a boiling broth and cook at low boil. As soon as they emerge, take out with a slotted spoon and lay on a dish.

Ravioli Tomato Sauce

ENERGY VALUE PER PORTION
CALORIE CONTENT 355 KCAL
SQUIRRELS 9.2 GRAM
FATS 27.1 GRAM
CARBOHYDRATES 19.1 GRAM
INGREDIENTS

- Saltto taste
- Butter 25 g
- Gruyere cheese 100 g
- Sugar 1 teaspoon
- Tomatoes 1.5 kg
- Onion 50 g
- Sunflower oil 3 tablespoons

COOKING INSTRUCTION 1 HOUR PRINT

1. Finely chop the onion. Peel the tomatoes and cut them into cubes. Cheese must be grated.

2. Heat the sunflower oil in a pan, add the onions and cook on low heat for 5 minutes until it becomes soft. Add the tomatoes and fry, crushing them with a spatula, for another 10 minutes. Let the mixture cool slightly, then transfer to a blender and mash. Add sugar and a pinch of salt.

3. Preheat the oven to 200 degrees. Put a little sauce in a fireproof dish, sprinkle with half the cheese. Place ravioli on top of the cheese and fill with the remaining sauce. Sprinkle with cheese and butter again. Bake for 20-30 minutes until they turn golden brown.

Cheese and Basil Ravioli

ENERGY VALUE PER PORTION
CALORIE CONTENT 774 KCAL
SQUIRRELS 33.1 GRAM
FATS 36,4 GRAM
CARBOHYDRATES 77.6 GRAM
INGREDIENTS

- Marjoram 1 stalk
- Wheat flour 400 g
- 4 eggs
- Ricotta cheese 200 g
- Pecorino cheese 100 g
- ½ beambasil
- Butter 50 g
- Parmesan Cheese 50 g
- Saltto taste
- Ground black pepperto taste

COOKING INSTRUCTION 43 MINUTES

1. For the dough, pour the flour up the slide on the desktop, in the center make a recess. In the recess, put eggs, 0.5 teaspoons of salt. Knead the dough until it becomes smooth and elastic. Cover with a towel and leave for half an hour in the refrigerator.

2. For the filling, knead the ricotta with a fork, add the grated pecorino, salt, pepper to taste, add the chopped basil.

3. Divide the dough into 2 parts and roll out 2 thin layers of 2 mm thick. Cut the dough into strips 5 cm wide (preferably with a round knife with cloves). Half the strips to put small portions of the filling, backing 3 cm.

4. Cover with the remaining strips of dough and cut into squares (the filling should be in the center of the squares). Put ravioli on a towel sprinkled with flour and leave for 10-15 minutes.

5. Boil 3 liters of salted water, put ravioli in boiling water and cook for 3-4 minutes. Arrange on plates, pour with melted butter, sprinkle with grated Parmesan and garnish with basil or marjoram leaves.

Bechamel sauce for ravioli

ENERGY VALUE PER PORTION
CALORIE CONTENT 338 KCAL
SQUIRRELS 8.5 GRAM
FATS 28.9 GRAM
CARBOHYDRATES 11.2 GRAM
INGREDIENTS

- Saltto taste
- Gruyere cheese 50 g
- Tomato paste 2 tablespoons
- Milk 500 ml
- Wheat flour 1 tablespoon
- 2 tablespoonsolive oil
- Butter 50 g

COOKING INSTRUCTION 45 MINUTES

1. Melt half the butter and vegetable in the bucket. Stir in the flour and cook, stirring, for 2 minutes. Pour the milk slowly while continuing to stir. Salt and cook, stirring, for 5 minutes. Add the tomato puree. Shuffle.

2. Preheat the oven to 200 degrees. Put ravioli in a fireproof dish and pour the sauce. Sprinkle with grated cheese and slices of cream. Bake for 20-30 minutes until the cheese has melted and turns into a delicious crust.

Ravioli with beets, cottage cheese and parmesan

ENERGY VALUE PER PORTION
CALORIE CONTENT 666 KCAL
SQUIRRELS 31.3 GRAM
FATS 14.8 GRAM
CARBOHYDRATES 103,2 GRAM
INGREDIENTS

- Water 2 tablespoons
- Chicken egg 3 pieces
- Wheat flour 500 g
- Beets 2 pieces
- Curd 100 g
- Nutmegpinch
- Grated Parmesan Cheese 100 g
- Saltpinch

- Ground black pepperto taste

COOKING INSTRUCTION 45 MINUTES

1. To fill the beets, wash, boil or bake in the oven until cooked, cool and grate on a coarse grater.
2. Put the beets in a fine sieve and squeeze, forcefully pressing it with a spoon.
3. Squeezed beets mixed with cottage cheese (cottage cheese should be dense) and grated parmesan.
4. Add salt, pepper and nutmeg. To stir thoroughly. The filling should be thick enough.
5. For the dough, break the eggs into the cup, add water, salt and sifted flour - knead the soft dough.
6. On a powdery surface, roll out the dough into 2 thin layers.
7. On one layer put 1 teaspoon of the filling at a small distance from each other.
8. Cover with a second layer of dough and squeeze places not occupied by the filling.
9. Cut the dough into squares.
10. It is unnecessary to cut and fasten the edges with a fork.
11. In a wide saucepan, boil slightly salted water, put ravioli and cook until they pop up.
12. Carefully transfer them to a dish with a slotted spoon.
13. Serve with butter or sour cream.

Ravioli with pesto and mushrooms

ENERGY VALUE PER PORTION
CALORIE CONTENT753KCAL
SQUIRRELS19,2GRAM
FATS32GRAM
CARBOHYDRATES98.9GRAM
INGREDIENTS

- Wheat flour 500 g
- Chicken egg 1 piece
- Olive oil 3 tablespoons
- Water ¾ cup
- Fresh spinach leaves 1 bunch
- Fresh mushrooms 500 g
- Onion 1 piece
- Butter 2 tablespoons
- Sour cream 2 tablespoons
- Saltto taste
- Ground black pepperto taste

COOKING INSTRUCTION 1 HOUR + 5 MINUTES

1. Knead the dough. Beat eggs with olive oil and water. Add salt. Grind the spinach in a mortar or in a blender and add to the egg mixture. Pour the sifted flour into this mixture gradually. Knead elastic and elastic dough, like dumplings. Ready to put off the dough for 30 minutes to rest.
2. Cook the minced meat. Finely chop the mushrooms and onions. Fry in butter, add sour cream or cream a little later. Pepper, salt and simmer for 10-15 minutes.
3. Blind ravioli. Divide the dough into two equal parts and roll it into thin layers. Spread the filling with a spoon at a distance of 4-5 cm from each other. Apply a second layer and firmly press the edges around the filling with your fingers. Cut them into squares or circles.
4. Cook ravioli in salted water for 5–7 minutes. Can be seasoned with olive oil and grated cheese.

Thin pizza dough

ENERGY VALUE PER PORTION
CALORIE CONTENT 200 KCAL
SQUIRRELS 4.6 GRAM
FATS 5,6 GRAM
CARBOHYDRATES 33.3GRAM

INGREDIENTS

- Wheat flour 175 g
- Saltto taste
- 1 tablespoonolive oil
- Dry yeast 1 teaspoon
- Water 125 ml

COOKING INSTRUCTION 1 HOUR

1. Combine flour, salt and yeast in a food processor. Combine oil and water in a jug. Without turning off the combine, pour in liquid and knead a homogeneous dough. Transfer to a table sprinkled with flour and knead the dough for 2-3 minutes.

2. Transfer the dough into a bowl and grease the outside with olive oil. Cover the bowl with cling film and place in a warm place for 40 minutes until the dough is doubled.

3. Knead the dough again for 1-2 minutes. Roll out the dough into a circle of 30 cm and put on a baking sheet. Squeeze 2 cm from the edge to make a crust and fill with the filling of your choice.

RISOTTO

Saffron risotto with porcini mushrooms

INGREDIENTS
- Arborio rice 200 g
- Ceps 120 g
- Parmesan Cheese 30 g
- Shallots 13 g
- Garlic 1 clove
- Thyme 1 g
- Parsley 3 g
- Butter 30 g
- Saffron 0.1 g
- Dry white wine 50 ml
- Olive oil 40 ml

COOKING INSTRUCTION 20 MINUTES

1. Cut shallots and garlic into a small cube and fry in olive oil for 2-3 minutes until the onions are clear.
2. Add rice and fry another 1 minute, pour dry white wine and evaporate until the smell of alcohol disappears.
3. Pour 3/4 of the rice with water, simmer, stirring continuously and adding hot water for 15 minutes.
4. Dice the ceps and sauté in olive oil for 2 minutes.
5. In the middle of the stewing process, add butter, salt and pepper to taste, saffron on the tip of the knife and continue to simmer, stirring constantly.
6. Add the fried mushrooms to rice 3 minutes before the end of cooking, evaporate water.
7. Put the risotto on a plate with a slide, sprinkle with finely chopped parsley and grated parmesan, garnish with a sprig of thyme and serve.

Chicken Breast Risotto

INGREDIENTS
- Arborio rice 120 g
- Onion 1 piece
- Garlic 1 clove
- Chicken fillet 500 g
- Dry white wine 70 ml
- Parmesan Cheese 40 g
- Saffronon the tip of a knife
- Saltto taste
- Ground black pepperto taste

COOKING INSTRUCTION 25 MINUTES

1. Dilute a pinch of saffron in 50 ml of boiling water. Onions, chop finely chopped garlic.
2. Fry onion, garlic, chicken in a non-stick pan without oil. Pour rice, add wine and evaporate for two to three minutes.
3. Pour in the saffron infusion and cook, stirring constantly. Add water as it evaporates and stir constantly.
4. Total rice should cook for 17 minutes. At 15 minutes, salt and pepper the risotto, add grated parmesan, mix, and serve.

Risotto with Asparagus

INGREDIENTS
- Fresh Asparagus 1 kg
- 4 tablespoonsolive oil

- Chicken stock 1 l
- Onion 1 head
- Rice for risotto 360 g
- Grated Parmesan Cheese 85 g
- Cream 3 tablespoons

COOKING INSTRUCTION 30 MINUTES

1. Wash the asparagus and cut off the tops.
2. Cook the asparagus stalks in boiling water for 8 minutes until soft. Drain and transfer into a chicken stock blender. Beat, pour into a frying pan, bring to a boil, and then lightly heat over low heat.
3. Cook the asparagus tops in boiling water for 1 minute. Drain and chill in ice water.
4. Heat the olive oil in a large pan, add the finely chopped onions and lightly fry. Add rice and reduce heat. Add salt and spices and mix well. Add a soup ladle of hot broth with asparagus and cook over medium heat, stirring constantly until the whole has evaporated, then add another soup broth and so on. Simmer for about 20 minutes until rice is cooked.
5. Add the parmesan and cream and gently stir the boiled asparagus. Serve hot.

Buckwheat Risotto

INGREDIENTS

- Buckwheat groats 120 g
- Eggplant 200 g
- Cream 10% 150 ml
- Dry white wine 150 ml
- Grated Parmesanto taste
- Dried thymepinch
- Dried oreganopinch
- Basil leavesto taste
- Black pepper peas 5 pieces
- Saltto taste
- Garlic 1 clove
- Olive oil 20 ml

COOKING INSTRUCTION 25 MINUTES

1. Heat olive oil in a pan with a thick bottom.
2. Cut the eggplant into cubes, chop the garlic finely.
3. Fry the garlic in a pan, add the eggplant. Fry for 5 minutes
4. Pour buckwheat, fry with eggplant, stirring.
5. Reduce the heat and add wine. Mix.
6. Once the liquid is absorbed, pour a glass of water into the pan. Mix.
7. Pound black pepper in a mortar. If you use coarse wet salt, it will be great to crush the pepper along with the salt.
8. Monitor the amount of liquid in the pan. Once absorbed, pour a glass of water. Let it boil for another 10 minutes.
9. Add salt with pepper, thyme, oregano.
10. Pour the cream, mix, hold for another 3 minutes and done.
11. Already in a bowl, sprinkle "risotto" with parmesan and garnish with basil leaves.

Risotto with vegetables, onions and carrots

INGREDIENTS

- Rice 200 g
- Onion 1 head
- Carrot 1 piece
- Sweet pepper 200 g
- Olive oil 3 tablespoons
- Canned Corn 150 g

- Saltto taste
- Greensto taste

COOKING INSTRUCTION 25 MINUTES

1. Rinse the rice in cold water until the water becomes clear. We put it in a pan, pour cold water, put on fire. Bring to a boil, salt (to taste), reduce the heat. Simmer for 12 minutes.
2. Cut the onion into half rings, carrots into small cubes. Fry in a pan in olive oil.
3. From the pepper we take out the core, rinse and cut into cubes.
4. Spread rice, canned corn, pepper in a pan with onions and carrots, mix everything thoroughly.
5. When serving, decorate with greens.

Motley vegetable risotto

INGREDIENTS

- Arborio rice ½ cup
- Pumpkin 200 g
- Green peas ½ cup
- Carrot 1 piece
- Leek 30 g
- Onion 1 head
- Brussels sprouts 60 g
- Green bell pepper ½ pieces
- Saffronon the tip of a knife
- Bay leaf 2 pieces
- Black pepper peasto taste
- 2 tablespoonsolive oil
- Vegetable broth1.2 l
- Garlic4 cloves

COOKING INSTRUCTION 1 HOUR

1. Cook the vegetable broth (carrots, turnips, kohlrabi leaves, celery root, onions and white cabbage with a pinch of coriander and two bay leaves for flavor), after the broth is ready, leave it on low heat so that it does not cool.
2. We throw washed arborio rice into the stew-pan, heat it for less than a minute and fill it with hot vegetable broth, throw the garlic cloves cut lengthwise and across, and mix thoroughly. As the broth is absorbed, pour more and mix, cook there until the rice is ready (about 20-30 minutes); in the middle of cooking, you can add saffron, slightly crumbling on top of rice and stirring.
3. Finely chop the onions and carrots in small cubes of 5x5 mm. Cut the pumpkin into cubes a little larger, cut the leek into small rings. 15 minutes before rice is cooked, we throw onions and carrots into the wok and simmer for 5 minutes over high heat, then we throw pumpkin and bell pepper (in my case it was dried), a little later we throw Brussels sprouts.
4. Stew until the pumpkins are ready. Add frozen green peas.
5. Once the rice is ready, mix everything together, if necessary, add more broth, leave to reach. After 10-15 minutes, the risotto is ready to serve. While serving, garnish with herbs or fresh vegetables (carrots or fresh bell peppers), sprinkle with lemon juice and olive oil.

Risotto with sea cocktail

INGREDIENTS

- Onions 100 g
- Rice 300 g
- Extra virgin olive oil 40 ml
- Dry white wine 200 ml
- Saffron 1 teaspoon
- Fish stock 1 l
- Saltto taste

- Seafood Cocktail 400 g

COOKING INSTRUCTION 1 HOUR 30 MINUTES

1. Onion finely chopped and sautéed in olive oil for 2-3 minutes. Then add the washed rice, cook another 2-3 minutes.
2. Pour white wine into the pan. Stirring, simmer the whole thing until the wine is completely evaporated.
3. When the wine has evaporated, add saffron, mix. Now one ladle (about 200 ml) is added to the rice fish broth. When the first soup ladle is almost completely evaporated, add the second, after the second - the third, etc., until the broth ends.
4. After about 15 minutes, the rice will be almost ready. We taste, if necessary, salt to taste.
5. Add a seafood cocktail to the rice (if you have a frozen cocktail, you must first thaw it at room temperature). Stir and cook over medium heat for about 5 minutes.

Risotto with salmon and dill

INGREDIENTS
- Zucchini 200 g
- Onion 1 head
- Green String Beans 200 g
- 2 tablespoonsolive oil
- Butter 15 g
- Dillto taste
- Saltto taste
- Ground black pepperto taste
- Rice 300 g
- Vegetable broth 1,299 l
- Salmon Fillet 600 g

COOKING INSTRUCTION 45 MINUTES PRINT

1. Vegetables - zucchini and beans - bake on the grill or in the oven. Cut into small pieces.
2. Salmon fillet can also be baked, but you can fry it in a small amount of olive oil in a pan. If you prefer lighter foods, you can boil the fish. Let the salmon cool, and then divide it into "flakes".
3. Finely chop the onion. Rinse the rice. Heat the olive oil in a large saucepan. Add the same slice of butter, melt and mix. Place chopped onions in a pan and fry until soft. Then add the rice and mix so that the whole rice is covered with butter.
4. Pour a little warmed broth into the pan, mix. Bring to a boil and stir until rice has absorbed the entire broth. Then add a little more broth and repeat until you use the whole broth.
5. Add salmon, vegetables and finely chopped dill to the pan with rice and mix well. Hold on the fire for another minute, salt and pepper to taste and serve.

Risotto with pear and gorgonzola

INGREDIENTS
- Butter 2 tablespoons
- Pear 2 pieces
- Sugar 1 tablespoon
- Onion 1 head
- Chicken broth 3 cups
- Arborio rice 1 cup
- White dry wine ½ cup
- Gorgonzola cheese 120 g

COOKING INSTRUCTION 35 MINUTES

1. In a deep pan, melt 1 tablespoon of butter. Add the pears and sugar chopped into small pieces and cook until the pears are caramelized. Put on a plate.
2. Bring the broth to a boil.

3. In the same pan, melt the remaining butter and fry the finely chopped onions until soft. Add rice and fry until translucent for 2-3 minutes.

4. Pour in the wine, then 0.5 cups of broth and cook until all the liquid has evaporated. Cook for about 20-30 minutes until the rice is soft, adding to the broth as you evaporate.

5. Add pear and gorgonzola and mix well6 until the cheese melts.

Risotto with marine reptiles

INGREDIENTS
- Arborio rice 280 g
- Seafood Cocktail 400 g
- Mussels 20 pieces
- Langoustines 4 pieces
- Tiger prawns 4 pieces
- Dry white wine320 ml
- Olive oil 12 tablespoons
- Onion 2 heads
- Fish broth 700 ml
- Chopped parsley 2 tablespoons
- Garlic 4 cloves
- Ground white pepperto taste
- Sea saltto taste
- Cayenne pepperon the tip of a knife

COOKING INSTRUCTION 1 HOUR

1. Peel and chop the onion into small cubes. Crush the garlic cloves with a knife.

2. Heat 11 tablespoons of olive oil until a characteristic odor appears. Reduce the heat to medium. Put the onion and lightly fry it with frequent stirring for 1 minute. Add the garlic.

3. Then pour in dry rice. You need to warm the rice with constant stirring until it slightly changes color.

4. Pour parsley and pour wine. Warm until alcohol evaporates.

5. Gently place the shrimp and lobster in the pan. Warm up, pour in a soup ladle of hot broth and add a sea cocktail and mussels.

6. The broth should be infused with ladles (total - 6-8 ladles). Each subsequent soup ladle should be infused when the previous portion has already been absorbed.

7. Add white pepper and salt. At the very end of cooking add a little cayenne pepper.

8. Remove large and fragile seafood and garlic from the risotto. Add 1 tablespoon of olive oil. Knead the risotto vigorously.

Pearl barley risotto with pumpkin

INGREDIENTS
- Pumpkin 200 g
- Leek 40 g
- Pearl barley 150 g
- Parmesan Cheese 40 g
- Butter 30 g
- Red onion 70 g
- Fennel 1 g
- Garlic 3 cloves
- Bay leaf 1 piece
- Vegetable broth 650 ml

COOKING INSTRUCTION 35 MINUTES

1. Peel the pumpkin from the peel and seeds and cut into a 1x1 cm slice, peel and chop the red onion, finely chop the leek, crush the garlic cloves, peel and chop coarsely; bring the broth to a boil.

2. Heat 1/3 butter in a deep pan and fry the fennel seeds in it over medium heat, stirring constantly, for 10 seconds.

3. Add 1 tablespoon of olive oil, garlic, leek and red onion and fry over high heat for 1 minute until the onions are golden.

4. Add pumpkin, bay leaf, salt, pepper and fry, stirring constantly, 2 minutes over medium heat; grate parmesan on a coarse grater.

5. Pour pearl barley into the pan and fry for 1 minute.

6. Pour the pearl barley with the hot broth so that the broth is on par with the cereal and simmer with a slight boil, stirring constantly and adding the broth as it evaporates for 30 minutes.

7. Put the remaining butter, mix; put the risotto in plates, sprinkle with parmesan and serve immediately.

Wild mushroom risotto

INGREDIENTS
- Rice bomb 200 g
- Frozen Forest Mushrooms 200 g
- Balsamic creamto taste
- 2 tablespoonsolive oil
- Dried basilpinch
- Chicken stock 1 l
- Ground dried garlicpinch

COOKING INSTRUCTION 30 MINUTES

1. Fry the mushrooms in olive oil until a yellow crust forms. Add a pinch of dried garlic to flavor.

2. Pour rice to the mushrooms and mix well. As the rice becomes clear, pour in white wine and simmer for about 2 minutes.

3. Chicken broth should be heated and poured into the rice in parts, as it is absorbed by the rice. Cook rice to al dente.

4. Grate the cheese and add to the rice with mushrooms, mix thoroughly, making the risotto creamy. Add basil and serve with balsamic cream and add a bright flavor to this dish.

Italian risotto with wild mushrooms

INGREDIENTS
- Shallots 2 pieces
- Garlic 2 cloves
- Dry white wine 500 ml
- Butter 50 g
- Rice for risotto 150 g
- Fresh mushrooms 100 g
- Olive oil 20 ml

COOKING INSTRUCTION 30 MINUTES

1. Heat olive oil in a large saucepan and add the garlic and shallots. Sauté for a while until soft.

2. Then add rice, pour in the remaining oil and add 0.5 bottles of white wine. Stew until tender.

3. In another pan, sauté the chopped mushrooms in olive oil until tender. Then add the butter.

4. Add a small amount of water to the pot with risotto and bring to a ready. Add the mushrooms and cook for some more time. Salt to taste and serve with a little fat cream.

Risotto with tomatoes (Cardinal)

INGREDIENTS
- Basil 14 g
- Olive oil 12 ml
- Spices 1 g
- Salt 4 g
- Carnaroli Rice 110 g

- Tomato Sauce 140 g
- Meat broth 250 ml
- Parmesan Cheese 25 g
- Butter 15 g
- Dry white wine 10 ml

COOKING INSTRUCTION 20 MINUTES

1. Fry the carnaroli rice with onions in a deep frying pan in olive oil.
2. Pour white wine, evaporate. Pour, evaporate.
3. Then gradually add the meat broth.
4. Cook on the senses. Rice should, of course, result in al dente. Everything rests on plus or minus a few minutes, the difference in volume, heat. Rice, we assume, turned out.
5. Add tomato sauce and butter.
6. Generously pour parmesan. The main thing is to stir, stir constantly, bringing everything to a cream state.
7. Then we throw fresh basil and still add a little broth. If you want, throw more cherry tomatoes in quarters.

Risotto with tartare

INGREDIENTS

- Rice for risotto 100 g
- Shallots 13 g
- Garlic 5 g
- Fresh thyme1 g
- Olive oil 40 ml
- Dry white wine 40 ml
- Butter 30 g
- Parmesan Cheese3 0 g
- Saltto taste
- Chicken stock 200 ml
- Ground black pepperto taste
- Parsley 2 g
- Marbled beef 80 g
- Quail egg1 piece

COOKING INSTRUCTION 30 MINUTES

1. Pour olive oil into a stewpan, add a clove of garlic and thyme and fry. Add finely chopped shallots (10 grams), fry, pour in rice, fry until rice is clear, pour in white wine, let it evaporate and pour hot chicken stock so that it covers rice by 2 cm. Cook on a low heat pouring the broth as needed. Add salt.
2. At the end of cooking add grated parmesan, butter and mix well. Add olive oil (30 grams) and black pepper.
3. Cut the meat into small cubes, add the finely chopped shallots and parsley, salt, add black pepper and olive oil.
4. Put the tartar through the mold into the center of the plate, make a small depression in the middle and release the yolk of the quail egg into it, lay the finished risotto around. Garnish with thin slices of parmesan.

Risotto with chanterelles, shallots and parmesan

INGREDIENTS

- Chicken broth 3 cups
- Salted butter 4 tablespoons
- Shallots 2 pieces
- Little chanterelles 450 g
- Saltto taste

- Freshly ground black pepperto taste
- Rice for risotto 1 cup
- Grated Parmesan 60 g

COOKING INSTRUCTION 30 MINUTES

1. Pour the broth into a saucepan and bring to a boil, make a small fire and keep it hot.

2. Melt half the butter in a small saucepan over high heat, add chopped shallots and sauté for 1 minute. Add the little chanterelles whole and fry until soft for 5 minutes. Salt and pepper and transfer to a bowl.

3. In the same saucepan, melt the remaining butter over medium heat, add rice, mix well and fry for 3 minutes. pour a glass of hot broth and cook, stirring, until the liquid evaporates. Cook by adding the broth for about 25 minutes until the rice is soft and creamy. Add mushrooms before pouring the last portion of the broth. Add the parmesan, check the amount of salt and serve immediately.

Pumpkin Risotto

INGREDIENTS
- Vegetable broth 8 glasses
- 5 tablespoonsolive oil
- Onion 1 head
- Pumpkin butternut squash 2 cups
- Arborio Rice 2 cups
- Dry white wine 1 cup
- Grated Parmesan cheese 120 g
- Chives 2 tablespoons
- Saltto taste

COOKING INSTRUCTION 1 HOUR

1. Peel the pumpkin of the skin and seeds and cut into small cubes to make 2 cups.

2. In a saucepan, bring the broth to a boil, make a very small fire and leave to warm.

3. In a large saucepan, heat 4 tablespoons of olive oil and add finely chopped onions and pumpkin. Sauté for 5 minutes until the onion is translucent.

4. Pour rice and fry, stirring, 1-2 minutes.

5. Then pour the wine and cook, stirring, until the wine has evaporated.

6. Pour a few soup ladles into the broth and cook over medium heat, stirring until the broth evaporates, then pour in another broth and continue cooking for 15–20 minutes until the rice is ready.

7. A few minutes before cooking, add the remaining oil, 0.3 cups of Parmesan and finely chopped chives. Salt and mix. Cook for a while longer until the risotto is creamy.

8. Serve by sprinkling with the remaining parmesan.

Arugula Risotto

INGREDIENTS
- Frozen Green Peas 500 g
- Chicken Broth 1.2 L
- Garlic 4 cloves
- Green onion 10 pieces
- Arborio rice 300 g
- Arugula150 g
- Sea saltto taste
- Ground black pepperto taste
- Vegetable oil 2 tablespoons
- Grated Parmesanto taste

COOKING INSTRUCTION 45 MINUTES

1. Boil 600 milliliters of chicken broth in a saucepan and boil slightly defrosted green peas in it for 5 minutes. Pour into a blender bowl and beat in a homogeneous mass. Then pour it back into the pan and add the remaining 600 milliliters of broth.

2. Peel and crush the garlic in a mortar, finely chop the green onion. Heat oil in a large pan and fry the garlic and onions for a minute.

3. Add rice and fry, stirring constantly, for another couple of minutes.

4. Pour a little pea broth with a ladle so that it covers the rice. Cook over low heat for 15 minutes, stirring slowly and adding more and more broth as needed. Season with salt and pepper. Before serving, sprinkle with grated Parmesan and garnish with arugula, as well as fresh vegetables or mushrooms fried in vegetable oil.

Chicken Risotto with Soy Sauce

INGREDIENTS
- Rice 200 g
- Chicken fillet 400 g
- Soy sauce 150 ml
- Dry white wine 150 ml
- 2 tablespoonsolive oil
- Garlic 3 pieces
- Onion 1 piece
- Greens1 bunch
- Ground black pepperpinch

COOKING INSTRUCTION 30 MINUTES

1. Cut the chicken into small pieces. Mix with soy sauce and finely chopped garlic. Pickle one hour.
2. Put the meat in the heated oil in a pan. Fry until cooked.
3. Rinse the rice so that there is no cloudy residue. Drain water from rice.
4. Cut the onion and fry it in oil until bright brown. Take out and discard the onion.
5. Pour rice into oil. Fry for 5 minutes.
6. Add the wine, simmer the rice in the wine, stirring until the wine evaporates.
7. Add a glass of water or meat broth. Cook, stirring, over medium heat for 15 minutes, adding water if necessary.
8. Salt, pepper rice to taste. Cover, let stand for 10-15 minutes.
9. Put rice on plates, put chicken on top, decorate with greens.
10. By adding grated cheese and a slice of butter in rice, we will make this dish more satisfying.

Summer risotto with herbs, feta and zucchini

INGREDIENTS
- 2 tablespoonsolive oil
- Garlic2 cloves
- Young zucchini 500 g
- Rice for risotto 350 g
- Basil leaves 25 g
- Vegetable broth 1.2 l
- Mint leaves 20 g
- Saltto taste
- Freshly ground black pepperto taste
- Feta cheese 100 g

COOKING INSTRUCTION 25 MINUTES

1. Heat the olive oil in a deep pan and add the thinly sliced zucchini. Cook over medium heat for 5 minutes until golden brown. Add chopped garlic, salt and pepper and cook for another minute. Add rice and stir for another 1 minute.
2. Bring the broth to a boil and add 1 ladle to the rice, stirring and adding the next, when the previous one has evaporated. Cook for 15-20 minutes, until the rice is soft and the consistency is creamy.
3. Remove from heat and add chopped basil and mint. Then add chopped feta and leave for 1 minute. Check the amount of salt and serve.

Mushroom risotto

INGREDIENTS

- Arborio rice 300 g
- Butter 100 g
- Onion 1 head
- Dry white wine 200 ml
- Chicken stock 1 l
- Champignons 300 g
- Saltto taste
- Saffronpinch

COOKING INSTRUCTION 25 MINUTES

1. Finely chop the onion and fry in a saucepan in butter until the onion starts to smell fried, add finely chopped mushrooms, fry them until they release water. Then pour rice into the stewpan and fry it together with onions and mushrooms for two minutes, stirring constantly.

2. Pour rice and onions with chicken stock and wine. Cook without a lid, stirring constantly. When the broth and wine are half-evaporated, add a tiny pinch of saffron and salt. While stirring, cook until rice is cooked. If the liquid boils too soon, add water, wine or broth.

Risotto with cream and sweet pepper

INGREDIENTS

- Rice 400 g
- Butter 100 g
- Sweet pepper 2 pieces
- Onion 1 head
- Garlic 4 cloves
- Vegetable broth 1.5 l
- Sherry 100 ml
- Cream 35% 100 ml
- Thyme 4 pieces
- Saltto taste
- Ground black pepperto taste

COOKING INSTRUCTION 20 MINUTES

1. Melt butter (80 g) in a deep frying pan and fry finely chopped onions on it. The bow should be completely soft and translucent. Pour rice and fry it for several minutes, stirring constantly. Add finely chopped garlic, mix, darken with rice, oil and onions; as soon as the garlic has practically dissolved in the mass of rice and onion and begins to emit its most characteristic of odors, pour dry sherry into the pan, mix with rice and vegetables and, removing the fire to a minimum, evaporate alcohol, stirring constantly.

2. As soon as the aroma exclusively reminds of the presence of sherry, pour a third of the broth into the pan, mix the contents of the pan so that the broth penetrates all the most secret minks, and cook rice over low heat, adding to the broth as it boils.

3. In the remaining butter, fry finely chopped and peeled seeds and other internal excesses. Peppers should become soft and start to smell fried.

4. Pour the peppers into a pan with a half-prepared risotto, salt, pepper, stir, add the broth and continue the same gimmick with cooking - stir, add the broth.

5. When the rice is almost ready, mix the cream into it. Turn off the heat and stir the contents of the pan for about a minute to achieve a creamy risotto consistency.

6. Serve sprinkled with thyme leaves.

Milanese risotto

INGREDIENTS

- Rice 400 g
- Chicken Broth 1.5 L
- Parmesan Cheese 50 g
- Onions 200 g
- Leek 100 g
- Garlic 2 cloves
- Saffronon the tip of a knife
- Tomatoes 100 g
- Butter 120 g
- Olive oil 50 ml
- Dry white wine 200 ml
- Parsley 20 g
- Saltto taste
- Ground black pepperto taste

COOKING INSTRUCTION 25 MINUTES

1. Dilute a pinch of saffron in 50 ml of boiling water. Chop onions, garlic and leek.
2. In a mixture of oils (100 g butter and 50 ml olive), fry the onions to an almost transparent softness, add garlic and leek and fry them until a garlic aroma appears. Leek will have time to become soft during this time. Add rice and fry it with vegetables for two to three minutes. Rice should thoroughly soak in butter.
3. Pour in a third of the available broth, white wine and cook rice, stirring constantly. As soon as the broth boils, the fire must be reduced. So that the liquid gurgles only slightly. Cook, stirring constantly and adding broth. After five minutes, pour saffron infusion into the rice and continue the story with stirring and topping the broth.
4. Fifteen minutes later, you can begin to try the rice, and as soon as it seems to you that it is almost ready, only somewhere inside the rice there is still a little bit of hardness, you need to salt and pepper the risotto, mix it with finely chopped parsley, add a little more a little broth, the rest of the butter (20 g), cook for two minutes, stirring occasionally.
5. Remove from heat and arrange in plates, adding to each a little salad of finely chopped fresh tomatoes mixed with olive oil and a little chopped onion, and sprinkle with grated Parmesan.

Chicken risotto

INGREDIENTS

- Arborio rice 350 g
- Onion 2 pieces
- Chicken fillet 400 g
- Canned Corn 200 g
- Yellow bell pepper 1 piece
- White semi-dry wine 200 ml
- Parmesan Cheese 100 g
- Chicken Broth 1.2 L
- Olive oil 30 ml
- Salt1 teaspoon
- Saffronon the tip of a knife
- Ground black pepper ¼ teaspoon

COOKING INSTRUCTION 1 HOUR

1. First, fry chopped onion in a small amount of oil, and then add small pieces of chopped chicken fillet.
2. When the chicken turns white, put in the pan cubes of yellow sweet pepper.

3. Mix, cook for a few minutes, then add saffron. I didn't have real saffron, but safflower (sometimes it is sold under the guise of saffron, but much cheaper). This spice can be put safely in a fairly large amount, but if there is a real saffron, it is better to put it.

4. Pour rice into the pan, salt, cook for 2-3 minutes.

5. Add wine in small portions while continuing to stir. When the wine is absorbed, we begin to pour in hot portions of the hot broth.

6. Add the corn.

7. Continue stirring and pouring the boiling broth in small portions.

8. When the rice is almost ready, try if there is enough salt, pepper.

9. Grate the parmesan to sprinkle the finished risotto at the end. Serve the risotto hot, sprinkled with parmesan.

Chanterelle Risotto

INGREDIENTS

- Rice 400 g
- Onions ½ heads
- Red onion 1 head
- Celery stalk 1 piece
- Chicken Broth 1.5 L
- Chanterelles 300 g
- Garlic 4 cloves
- Parsley 20 g
- Cream 100 ml
- Butter 100 g
- Olive oil 50 ml
- Saltto taste
- Ground black pepperto taste

COOKING INSTRUCTION 30 MINUTES

1. Finely chop the onion and celery and fry in a mixture of olive and butter. After the vegetables are softened, add the chanterelles (200 g), after cutting them. Fry chanterelles until cooked (the readiness is determined by taste: mushrooms must be thoroughly stewed, and onions and other vegetables should not be burned; usually, the juice released from the mushrooms is enough to prevent such a development of events, but if suddenly it was not enough, add a little a little oil or broth), then pour rice. Fry rice with mushrooms and vegetables for a couple of minutes, so that the rice absorbs mushroom, vegetable juices and oil. Then pour in a third of the broth, salt, pepper and leave over low heat, stirring constantly and, if necessary, pouring the broth in small portions.

2. Meanwhile, in another pan, interrupting to stir the rice, fry the remaining chanterelles (without slicing them) in a mixture of olive and butter. When the chanterelles stop giving water and begin to confidently fry, toss finely chopped garlic, salt, pepper, hold on fire for a couple of minutes, and then season with finely chopped parsley.

3. When the rice is ready, turn off the heat and pour the cream, interfering them with a spatula in the rice mass. Serve risotto garnished with fried chanterelles.

Risotto with mussels and shrimp

INGREDIENTS

- Rice 400 g
- Mussels 500 g
- Tomatoes 200 g
- Shrimp 300 g
- Red onions ½ heads
- Bay leaf 1 piece
- Parsley 20 g
- Dry white wine 200 ml

- Dry Martini 50 ml
- Olive oil 50 ml
- Vegetable broth 1.5 l
- Butter 20 g
- Lemon 1 piece
- Thyme1 piece
- Black pepper peas 5 pieces
- Ground white pepperto taste
- Saltto taste

COOKING INSTRUCTION 20 MINUTES

1. Fry finely chopped onions in a saucepan in butter until soft. Pour a glass of wine into a saucepan, toss a sprig of thyme, black peppercorns, bay leaf and pour mussels. Salt, if the mussels are fresh, do not. Fresh mussels have enough natural salinity.

2. Cover the pan with a lid and cook the contents over medium heat until the mussels open - about three minutes. As soon as the mussels open, throw to them in the company, peeled shrimp, chopped tomatoes, chopped parsley, pepper, stir and remove from heat.

3. In another stewpan, heat the olive oil and fry the rice on it so that it is saturated with oil, and pour a third of the available broth into the stewpan.

4. Once the broth boils, reduce the temperature and cook, stirring constantly and adding the broth as it boils. Together with one of the injections of the broth, you need to pour a glass of martini. When the rice is almost ready, it must be salted.

5. Then add a pinch of parsley, lemon juice and dump everything from the pan - mussels, shrimp and onions, along with the broth, in which all this was cooked. Mix gently and immediately remove from heat.

Risotto with porcini mushrooms and parsley

INGREDIENTS
- Rice 500 g
- Ceps 350 g
- Garlic 2 cloves
- 5 tablespoonsolive oil
- Butter 50 g
- Parsley 1 bunch
- Mushroom broth 1 l
- Grated Parmesanto taste
- Saltto taste

COOKING INSTRUCTION 40 MINUTES

1. Rinse the mushrooms thoroughly and chop finely. Finely grate the garlic, toss it in a pan with olive oil, stew for half a minute - then add the mushrooms and fry over high heat. When the mushrooms are ready, add salt and finely chopped parsley (half a bunch).

2. Meanwhile, put a piece of butter in another pan and add the washed rice, fry it until transparent and until all the butter has been absorbed. Then gradually pour the broth over the ladle, not forgetting to mix. It is important not to forget: while cooking rice - do not let the mushrooms cool, keep them warm.

3. When the rice is half ready, add the mushrooms (1/2 serving). Then continue to pour the broth. When the rice is finally ready, add a piece of butter, grated parmesan and the remaining parsley.

4. Distribute on plates, put the remaining mushrooms in the center of each plate, pour over the juice released during frying. Separately serve grated parmesan.

Risotto with porcini mushrooms and cream

INGREDIENTS
- Onion 1 head
- Carnaroli rice 500 g
- Garlic 4 cloves

- Fresh mushrooms 500 g
- Dry white wine 200 ml
- Butter 50 g
- Olive oil 50 ml
- Chicken Broth 1.5 L
- Parmesan Cheese 50 g
- Cream 20% 100 ml
- Saltto taste

COOKING INSTRUCTION 30 MINUTES

1. Onion finely chopped, chopped garlic. In a deep skillet (stewpan with a thick bottom), heat olive oil and a slice of butter.

2. First, fry the onions until transparent. Pour rice into sauteed onions, stir constantly (for several minutes) then add garlic and mix thoroughly.

3. Add mushrooms, stir for 2–4 minutes. Add white dry wine to the risotto. Stir continuously. After a few minutes add chicken stock. It should be infused in small doses, the first dose is 2 ladles, then, as one evaporates, one ladle.

4. During the preparation of the risotto, the broth should be kept in a boiling state, i.e. very heated, but not boiling. After 15 minutes of cooking, rice should be tried. He must be able to al dente. Add a little salt to the risotto.

5. Pour the cream into a bowl, grate the cheese on a fine grater, mix. Remove the risotto from the heat and carefully mix in the cream cheese mixture. Allow to stand for several minutes, then serve.

Meat risotto

INGREDIENTS

- Red onion 2 heads
- Celery 1 stalk
- Ground beef 250 g
- Carrot 1 piece
- Chicken liver 2 pieces
- Dry red wine ½ cup
- Tomato paste 100 g
- Arborio Rice ½ kg
- Butter 6 tablespoons
- Olive oil 125 ml
- Ground red pepperto taste
- Saltto taste
- Grated Parmesanto taste
- Ground black pepperto taste
- 6 cupchicken broth

COOKING INSTRUCTION 50 MINUTES

1. Chop red onion, celery stalk and carrots.

2. On medium heat, heat the risotto pan (deep pan or low wide pan), pour the olive oil and add half the butter. Add the chopped vegetables and stir, cook for about 3 minutes or until the onions are golden.

3. In parallel, in a separate pan, put the broth to warm up. In the process of preparing the dish, it is advisable to keep the broth on a very quiet fire and add to the risotto as warmed up.

4. Add minced meat to vegetables and cook for about 3 minutes.

5. Add 1 cup hot chicken stock, finely chopped chicken liver, wine, tomato paste, red and black pepper, and salt. Mix the INGREDIENTS well while chopping the minced meat. Cook over low heat for 10 minutes.

6. Add rice and cook, stirring frequently to al dente for about 25 minutes. As the liquid absorbs, add a little chicken stock (about 0.5 cup at a time). You should use the whole chicken stock (you can add more stock or red wine as needed).

7. When the rice is ready, turn off the heat, add the remaining butter, mix.

8. Serve the dish hot, sprinkled with parmesan.

Chicken and Parmesan Risotto

INGREDIENTS

- Chicken 1 kg
- Celery stalk 1 piece
- Onion 2 pieces
- Carrot 1 piece
- Butter 100 g
- Dry white wine 200 ml
- Arborio rice 200 g
- Parmesan Cheese 50 g
- Saltto taste
- Ground black pepperto taste

COOKING INSTRUCTION 1 HOUR 30 MINUTES

1. Separate chicken from bones. Dice the meat. Finely chop one onion.

2. Put chicken bones, celery, carrots and a whole onion in a pan, pour 1.5 liters of water, salt and pepper and bring to a boil. Reduce heat and cook for 30 minutes. Strain the broth and pour 500 ml into a clean pan. Put the broth on the fire and heat so that it boils softly.

3. Melt 65 grams of butter in another pan, add onion and chicken and cook over low heat, stirring for 10 minutes, until the chicken turns golden brown. Salt, pepper and add wine. Cook for 12–15 minutes until the liquid evaporates.

4. Pour the rice and cook, stirring, for 2 minutes until the rice becomes clear. Add the broth to cover the whole rice, and cook, stirring, until the liquid is completely absorbed. Add broth again, continue cooking, stirring occasionally. Do not pour the next portion of the broth until the previous one is completely absorbed.

5. When the whole broth is absorbed and the risotto is almost ready (it will take about 20 minutes), remove the pan from the heat and stir in the remaining butter and grated parmesan. Cover, wait 5-7 minutes, then serve.

Salmon Risotto

INGREDIENTS

- Trout 150 g
- Arborio rice 200 g
- Shallots 50 g
- Parmesan Cheese 50 g
- Butte r30 g
- Dill 5 g
- Lemon 40 g
- Garlic 1 clove
- Vegetable broth 650 ml
- Dry white wine 70 ml
- Olive oil 15 ml

COOKING INSTRUCTION 25 MINUTES PRINT

1. Peel and finely chop the onion and garlic, grate the parmesan on a fine grater; bring the vegetable stock to a boil.

2. Heat olive and 1/3 butter in a deep frying pan and fry the onions over medium heat until transparent for 1 minute, add garlic and fry for another 10 seconds, pour rice and fry constantly stirring for another 1 minute.

3. Pour in 70 ml of dry white wine, let the wine evaporate, pour the hot broth in the rice so that the broth is on par with the rice and simmer with gentle boiling, stirring constantly and adding the broth as it evaporates for 18 minutes.

4. Squeeze lemon juice, chop dill; cut the fish into strips 5 mm wide, salt, pepper, sprinkle with lemon juice.

5. Add the remaining butter to the risotto, stir it vigorously, slightly salt, add 1/3 of the parmesan, mix.

6. Add the fish to the risotto, stir and simmer for 30 seconds.

7. Arrange the risotto in plates, sprinkle with dill, remaining Parmesan and serve.

Chicken and Mushroom Risotto

INGREDIENTS

- Champignons 400 g
- Chicken fillet 200 g
- Jasmine Thai rice 200 g
- Red bell pepper 1 piece
- Onion 1 head
- Garlic 3 cloves
- Cherry Tomatoes 6 pieces
- Tomato paste 1 tablespoon
- Dry white wine 2 tablespoons
- Grated gingeron a knife tip

COOKING INSTRUCTION 40 MINUTES

1. Cook rice until 2/3 of the readiness.

2. Chicken fillet cut into small cubes (1–2 cm side), fry until tender in a large preheated pan or in a saucepan with vegetable oil (this will be the main pan, the whole dish will reach it ready).

3. Continuing to fry the chicken, chop the onion into small cubes, chop the garlic finely or squeeze. Fry the onions and garlic together in a preheated pan with vegetable oil until golden brown, add to the chicken.

4. Chop the pepper into small cubes, cut the tomatoes into 4 pieces each, fry in another pan with the addition of tomato paste, add to the main pan.

5. Cut the mushrooms into slices, fry in any oil until golden brown.

6. Combine everything (including rice), add salt, pepper, ginger powder to taste.

7. Cover, bring to readiness within 5-7 minutes.

8. Serve alone or with light sauce (Thousand Islands, for example).

Shrimp risotto with white wine

INGREDIENTS

- 5 cupchicken broth
- Dry white wine ¾ cup
- Butter 6 tablespoons
- Garlic paste 2 teaspoons
- Red pepper flakes ¼ teaspoon
- Onions 200 g
- Shrimp 230 g
- Arborio rice 1.5 cups
- Chopped parsley 2.5 tablespoons

COOKING INSTRUCTION 30 MINUTES

1. In a saucepan, mix the broth and 0.25 glasses of wine and bring to a boil. Maintain a light boil.

2. Melt 2 tablespoons butter in a skillet over medium heat. Add half the garlic and red pepper, then the shrimp. Cook for 2 minutes until the shrimp begins to change color. Add the remaining wine and cook another 2 minutes. Drain the shrimp while preserving the juices.

3. Melt the remaining butter in a deep frying pan over medium heat. Add finely chopped onions and the remaining garlic. Strain for 4 minutes until the onion is golden. Add rice and stir for 2 minutes. Then add 2 cups of hot broth and cook, stirring constantly, until the liquid evaporates. Then add 1 cup of broth and cook like this, constantly pouring the broth for about 20 minutes, until the rice is soft. Then, add the shrimp juice left and cook for another 5 minutes. Remove from heat.

4. Stir in shrimp and 2 tablespoons of parsley. Salt and pepper. Put in plates and sprinkle with the remaining parsley.

Risotto with mushrooms and parmesan

INGREDIENTS
- Round rice 2 cups
- Chicken stock 1 l
- Onion 1 piece
- Garlic 2 cloves
- Fresh mushrooms ¼ g
- Parmesan cheeseto taste
- Vegetable oilto taste

COOKING INSTRUCTION 50 MINUTES

1. Heat oil in a pan with a thick bottom, add finely chopped onions and garlic, mushrooms, mix. As soon as the onion begins to fry, add rice, mix and reduce heat.
2. When the rice becomes clear, pour in the hot broth in portions, stirring constantly, until the liquid is absorbed. Serve immediately, sprinkled with grated cheese.

Barley Risotto

INGREDIENTS
- Pearl barley 450 g
- Orange zest 1 teaspoon
- Chicken broth 400 ml
- Thyme 1 stalk
- Butter 30 g
- Grated Parmesan 60 g
- Salttaste
- Ground black peppertaste

COOKING INSTRUCTION 35 MINUTES

1. Cook the barley in salted water until half cooked, for twenty to twenty-five minutes. Fold in a colander and rinse with cold water so that the cereal is not prepared by internal heat.
2. Transfer the barley to a large stewpan, add the broth, fresh zest and finely chopped thyme leaves. Simmer on low heat, stirring constantly, until the whole broth is absorbed - it takes about five minutes.
3. Stir in grated parmesan and butter in the risotto, salt and pepper to taste - and serve hot.

Mushroom risotto

INGREDIENTS
- Rice 300 g
- Onion 1 head
- Dry white wine 50 ml
- Dried porcini mushrooms100 g
- Butter 100 g
- Shallots 1 head
- Hard cheese 100 g
- Bay leaf 1 piece
- Thyme ¼ beam
- Saltto taste
- Ground black pepperto taste

COOKING INSTRUCTION 40 MINUTES

1. In a deep saucepan, fry the onions in butter.
2. Add rice, salt, pepper, bay leaf, thyme to the onion, add water, close the lid and cook over low heat for about 20 minutes.
3. Dried porcini mushrooms soak for an hour in warm water, then fry together with shallots in butter.

4. Combine the mushrooms with rice, add wine, grated cheese, the remaining butter, salt and pepper. To mix everything.

Risotto with Chicken, Vegetables and Parmesan

INGREDIENTS

- Butter 100 g
- Chicken fillet 300 g
- Saltto taste
- Ground black pepperto taste
- Onion 1 piece
- Rice 350 g
- Meat broth 3 cups
- Celery 2 Stalks
- Red bell pepper 1 piece
- Tomatoes 1 piece
- Carrot 1 piece
- Parmesan Cheese 100 g
- Basil 4 stalks

COOKING INSTRUCTION 1 HOUR

1. Wash, dry the chicken fillet, cut into small cubes. Melt half the butter in a thick-bottomed pan. Fry the chicken until golden brown, slightly salt, pepper. Simmer for 10-15 minutes, put in a separate plate and set aside.

2. Peel the onion, chop finely, put in the pan in which the chicken was fried. Stir fry over low heat until transparent. Rinse, dry, adding to the pan, mix well and let it warm up along with onions and oil.

3. Boil the broth in a separate pan, reduce the heat after boiling, do not remove the pan from the heat. When the rice becomes glassy, pour it with a small amount of hot broth, mix, allow the broth to completely absorb.

4. Wash, pepper, celery, tomato, carrots, peel and cut into small cubes, together with the fried chicken fillet, put on rice, then pour the remaining broth. Salt, pepper.

5. Add heat, cover and simmer, stirring occasionally and adding hot broth as necessary. Shortly before cooking, add the remaining oil, 2/3 of the grated cheese and finely chopped basil, mix. When serving, sprinkle with the remaining cheese.

Risotto with arugula and spinach

INGREDIENTS

- Rice 400 g
- Arugula 300 g
- Spinach 300 g
- Red onion 1 head
- Ginger 20 g
- Dry Martini 250 ml
- Olive oil 50 ml
- Vegetable broth 1.5 l
- Chili pepper ½ pieces
- Lime ½ pieces
- Parsley 20 g
- Thyme 1 piece
- Sugar 15 g
- Lemon ½ pieces
- Ground white pepperto taste
- Saltto taste

COOKING INSTRUCTION 20 MINUTES

1. Finely chop the ginger and onion and fry in olive oil. When the vegetables are soft, pour in rice, lightly fry it so that it is saturated with the aromas of vegetables and oil, then pour in the martini, mix, remove the heat so that the liquid gurgles slightly, and cook, stirring constantly, until the martini is completely evaporated.

2. Then pour in a third of the broth and continue cooking, constantly stirring and adding new portions of the broth as the liquid boils. During the second dose of the broth supplement, throw thyme leaves torn from a twig into a saucepan, salt and pepper.

3. When the rice is almost ready (here, as usual, you have to use your own taste), add sugar, finely chopped chili peppers and parsley, squeeze the juice of half lime and lemon, as well as arugula and spinach, after tearing them into small pieces. Boil the risotto, stirring, until the greens lose all their elastic qualities.

Garlic and tomato barley risotto

INGREDIENTS
- Cilantro (coriander) leavesto taste
- Pearl barley ½ cup
- 1 teaspoonolive oil
- Tomatoes 3 pieces
- Garlic 1 clove
- Basil 1 teaspoon
- Red pepper flakes ¼ teaspoon
- Tomato paste 2 tablespoons
- Sugar ½ teaspoon
- Saltto taste
- Vegetarian feta cheeseto taste

COOKING INSTRUCTION 1 HOUR

1. Add oil to the pan and, once warmed, add chopped garlic. Cook until the garlic is golden.

2. Add barley, tomatoes, basil, tomato paste, red pepper, salt and sugar with a cup of hot water. Stir and cook for 40-50 minutes, stirring from time to time to avoid sticking cereals, and pouring hot water when necessary, because barley should be covered with water.

3. When the risotto is ready, season to taste and arrange in bowls. Sprinkle feta cheese and cilantro on top. Serve the dish hot.

Chicken and Vegetable Risotto

INGREDIENTS
- Rice 350 g
- Chicken fillet 300 g
- Butter 75 g
- Meat broth 700 ml
- Olive oil 15 ml
- Onion 2 pieces
- Carrot 1 piece
- Tomatoes 2 pieces
- Sweet pepper 2 pieces
- Ground corianderto taste
- Saltto taste
- Ground black pepperto taste

COOKING INSTRUCTION 40 MINUTES

1. Cut the chicken into a small cube. We heat the pan with the addition of butter. Fry the chicken until golden brown.

2. Cut carrots, tomatoes and bell peppers. Cut the onion rings. Fry the onion in olive oil in a deep pan with a thick bottom.

3. Add rice for risotto to the pan. Mix. Pour in a little chicken stock. Stir until liquid is absorbed. We continue to pour the broth in portions, stirring constantly, for 15 minutes. 5 minutes before cooking, add coriander, carrots, tomato and bell pepper. Salt, pepper.
4. Spread rice with vegetables on a plate. Add the chicken.

Salads

Pomegranate Parsley Salad

Servings: 4
Preparation time: 15 minutes
INGREDIENTS:

- Two cucumbers, diced
- One minced garlic clove
- 1 ½ Cups chopped parsley
- Two green onions, chopped
- Salt Black pepper
- One pomegranate, seeded
- One juiced lemon

Instructions:

1. In a bowl, mix well all **INGREDIENTS**.
2. Serve.

Nutrition Value: Calories: 63 Fat: 0.4g Protein: 2.2g **CARBOHYDRATES**: 15.5g 37.

Raw Cauliflower Tomato Salad

Servings: 4
Preparation time: 15 minutes
INGREDIENTS:

- One head cauliflower, chopped
- Two tbsp lemon juice
- 2 Cups cherry tomatoes, halved
- Two tbsp chopped parsley
- Salt Black pepper
- Two tbsp pine nuts

Instructions:

1. Combine the cauliflower, lemon juice, parsley and cherry tomatoes in a bowl.
2. Add seasoning and mix well then top with pine nuts.
3. Serve.

Nutrition Value:Calories: 64 Fat: 3.3g Protein: 2.8g **CARBOHYDRATES**: 7.9g

Roasted Eggplant Salad

Servings: 6
Preparation time: 45 minutes
INGREDIENTS:

- Three eggplants, peeled and cubed
- One tsp basil
- Three tbsp extra virgin olive oil
- One tsp oregano
- Salt
- Black pepper
- 2 Cups cherry tomatoes, halved
- One tsp thyme
- One red onion, sliced

- Two tbsp chopped parsley

Instructions:

1. Preheat the oven at 350F.
2. Season the eggplants with salt, oregano, basil, thyme, pepper, and olive oil.
3. Spread them in a baking tray then bake for half an hour and transfer in a bowl.
4. Add the remaining **INGREDIENTS** and serve.

Nutrition Value: Calories: 148 Fat: 7.7g Protein: 3.5g **CARBOHYDRATES**: 20.5g

Tuscan Cabbage Salad

Servings: 4
Preparation time: 20 minutes
INGREDIENTS:

- One head cabbage, shredded
- One sliced red onion
- ½ Cup chopped parsley
- One red pepper, chopped
- One sliced green bell pepper
- Salt and pepper to taste
- One sliced yellow bell pepper
- Two tbsp apple cider vinegar
- 2 oz. pancetta, diced

Instructions:

1. Mix all **INGREDIENTS** in a bowl except the pancetta.
2. Cook the pancetta in a pan until it becomes crispy then once it cools stir it into the salad.
3. Serve and enjoy.

Nutrition Calories: 164 Fat: 6.5g Protein: 8.9g **CARBOHYDRATES**: 19.0g

Fish Salad

Serves 3
Prep time 5 minutes
INGREDIENTS

- 2 six-ounce cans tuna packed in water, Drained
- ½ cup Sliced celery
- ½ cup Sliced red grapes
- ¼ Thinly sliced red onion
- 2 tablespoons
- Sliced Greek Kalamata olives
- 1 tablespoon Chopped fresh oregano
- 2 tablespoons Chopped flat-leaf parsley
- 2 tablespoons Chopped fresh basil
- 2 tablespoons
- Lemon juice
- Salt and freshly ground pepper, to taste
- 1 tablespoon Olive oil
- 2 medium tomatoes, sliced

Directions

1. Combine all **INGREDIENTS** except for tomatoes in a medium bowl and toss gently.
2. Serve salad over the tomatoes and some dark greens.

Chickpeas and Eggplant Salad

Serves 4
Prep time 5 minutes
Cook Time 20 minutes
INGREDIENTS
- 1 garlic clove skinned and bashed
- 1 large eggplant chopped up into cubes
- 1 can of well-drained chickpeas
- 1 teaspoon of paprika
- 4 tablespoons of extra virgin olive oil
- Pepper and sea salt for seasoning
- Parsley leaves

Directions
1. Take a large sauté pan and heat the olive oil. Pour in the mashed garlic and heat till brown.
2. Add the eggplant then stir well till it is well coated with the oil.
3. Reduce heat and let it steam so that the vegetables cook slowly for about 15 minutes.
4. Keep stirring occasionally till cooked.
5. Once the eggplant is cooked and turns a nice brown color, pour in the paprika and chickpeas, then stir well and let it simmer.
6. Add salt and pepper to taste then simmer for a couple more minutes and then serve.

Pasta Salad

Serves 3
Prep time 5 minutes
Cook Time 25 minutes
INGREDIENTS
- 8 oz. multigrain farfalle
- 2 tsps. olive oil
- 1 lemon – Zest & juice
- 13.5 oz. artichoke hearts
- 8 oz. mozzarella cheese, freshly chopped
- ¼ cup chopped Red bell pepper, roasted
- ¼ cup freshly chopped parsley
- ½ cup frozen peas

Directions
1. Prepare the pasta according to package directions (omit fat and salt). Combine the zest, juiced lemon, and oil in a mixing container.
2. Drain and chop the artichoke. Add it and the rest of the fixings (cheese, parsley, and peppers). Toss well.
3. Add the peas to a colander. Pour the pasta and water over it when it's done. Shake to drain (don't run water over).
4. Add to the mixture and toss. Serve and enjoy at room temperature or warmed.

LEMON ROASTED POTATOES
Serves 4
Prep time 10 minutes
Cook time 30 minutes
INGREDIENTS
- 2 pounds Gold Potatoes
- ¼ cup Olive Oil
- 2 teaspoons Salt

- 1 tablespoon Garlic Powder
- 1 teaspoon Freshly Ground Pepper
- 1 Lemon
- 1 tablespoon Dried Oregano

Directions
1. Preheat the oven to 400°F.
2. Peel and wash the five-pounds of potatoes. Cut them into quarters. Spread the cut potatoes in the pan and into an even layer.
3. Juice the lemon, pouring it over the potato layer. Cut the peel into small pieces and add.
4. Add the olive oil, garlic powder, oregano, and salt and pepper to the pan, stirring gently. Bake for about 25-30 minutes, turning two times.
5. Potatoes will be ready when outsides are crispy, but insides are tender. Garnish entree with parsley.

Crispy Lentil Energy Bites

Serves 5
Prep time 10 minutes
Cook Time 30 minutes
INGREDIENTS
- ½ cup dry green lentils
- ½ tbsp. extra-virgin coconut oil, melted
- 1 tsp cinnamon
- 1 tsp coconut flour
- 1/8 tsp sea salt
- 2 cups dry quick oats
- ¼ cup unsweetened coconut, shredded
- ¼ cup pumpkin seeds
- ¼ organic dark chocolate chips
- ½ cup organic peanut butter
- ½ cup honey or maple syrup

Directions
1. Preheat your oven to 400°F and line a baking sheet with parchment paper. Rinse lentils and transfer them to a small saucepan.
2. Cover them with 2 cups of water and bring to a boil. Lower heat to medium and simmer for 15 minutes.
3. Drain lentils and transfer them to a small mixing bowl. Stir in the coconut oil and coat the lentils. Sprinkle with cinnamon, coconut flour and sea salt and stir well.
4. Spread lentils evenly onto lined baking sheet and bake for 15 minutes, stirring after halfway and keep an eye on them if they start to burn.
5. Set the lentils aside to cool. Meanwhile, in a large mixing bowl, stir together the oats, seeds, coconut and chocolate chips.
6. Add in crispy lentils, then the peanut butter and honey/maple syrup and stir well again. Roll into tablespoon sized balls and refrigerate for 30 minutes Serve and enjoy!

Easy Greek Summer Salad

Servings 4
Preparation 15 minutes
INGREDIENTS:
- Sun dried tomatoes - 1 4 cup, chopped
- Cucumber - 1, sliced
- Tomatoes - 1 lb., cubed

- Parsley - 1 4 cup, chopped
- Black olives - 1 2 cup
- Red onion – 1, sliced
- Salt and pepper - to taste
- Balsamic vinegar - 1 tbsp.
- Extra virgin olive oil - 2 tbsp.

Directions:
1. Take a separate bowl and mix together the tomatoes, cucumber, onion, parsley and black olives.
2. Sprinkle in a small amount of salt and pepper to suit your taste and then add olive oil and vinegar.
3. When all the **INGREDIENTS:** are combined, the salad is ready to eat.

Super Simple Mediterranean Salad

Servings 6
Preparation Time 20 minutes
INGREDIENTS:
- Red onion - 1, sliced
- Cilantro - 1 4 cup, chopped
- Almonds - 1 4 cup, sliced
- Parsley - 1 2 cup, chopped
- Tomatoes - 1 pound, sliced
- Fennel bulb - 1, sliced
- Cucumber - 1, sliced
- Lemon - 1, juiced
- Extra virgin olive oil - 2 tbsp.
- Balsamic vinegar - 1 tbsp.
- Oregano - 1 tsp., dried
- Salt and pepper - to taste

Directions:
1. Mix all of the above INGREDIENTS: (except salt and pepper) in a large salad bowl.
2. Add salt and pepper to suit your taste and gently stir together.
3. Serve salad as soon as mixed for best freshness.

Mediterranean Quick Salad

Servings 6
Preparation time 20 minutes
INGREDIENTS:
- Red bell pepper - 1, cored and diced
- Cucumber - 1, diced
- Cannellini beans - 1 can, drained
- Garlic clove - 1, chopped
- Red wine vinegar - 2 tbsp.
- Cherry tomatoes - 1 cup, halved
- Parsley - 1 2 cup, chopped
- Red onion - 1, sliced
- Almonds - 1 tbsp.
- Pine nuts - 2 tbsp.
- Salt and pepper - to taste

Directions:
1. In a large salad bowl, mix all **INGREDIENTS:** except nuts (almonds and pine nuts) and salt and pepper.
2. Season with salt and pepper to suit your taste and then mix again.

3. Sprinkle almonds and pine nuts on top. Eat right away.

Easy Grilled Chicken Salad

Servings 4
Preparation and Cooking time 30 minutes
INGREDIENTS:
- Chicken fillets - 2
- Extra virgin olive oil - 2 tbsp.
- Dried basil - 1 tsp.
- Oregano - 1 tsp.
- Salt and pepper - to taste
- Olive oil - 2 tbsp.
- Arugula - 2 cups of leaves
- Cherry tomatoes - 1 cup, halved
- Green olives - 1 4 cup
- Cucumber - 1, sliced
- Lemon - 1, juiced

Directions:
1. Mix all above INGREDIENTS: (except chicken, salt, pepper, oregano, basil and olive oil) in a large salad bowl and set aside.
2. Season the chicken with salt, pepper, oregano and basil then drizzle it with olive oil.
3. Sprinkle oregano, basil, salt and pepper onto chicken fillets evenly and then drizzle olive oil over fillets.
4. Put chicken fillets into a skillet over medium heat and cook until browned and cooked through.
5. Cut chicken into strips or dice. Add chicken to the other **INGREDIENTS:** and stir together.
6. Season with salt and pepper to suit your taste. Salad is best when served fresh.

Veggie Polenta Salad

Servings 4
Preparation and Cook time 40 minutes
INGREDIENTS:
- Polenta - 1 cup
- Water – 1 ¼ cups
- Tomatoes - 2, sliced
- Zucchini - 1 2 cup, sliced
- Eggplants - 2, sliced
- Dried basil - 1 tsp.
- Extra virgin olive oil - 2 tbsp.
- Balsamic vinegar - 2 tbsp.
- Dried oregano - 1 tsp.
- Salt and pepper - to taste

Directions:
1. Add a pinch of salt and the water to a sauce pan and heat to boiling.
2. Pour polenta into the boiling water and stir, cooking for about 3 minutes.
3. Remove from heat and pour polenta onto a square pan, smoothing the mixture to even it out.
4. Set aside until well cooled and then cut into small squares. Grill zucchini, eggplant and tomatoes and then put in a large bowl, adding the polenta cubes.
5. Mix in oil, vinegar, salt, pepper oregano and basil. Enjoy this fresh salad right away.

Baked Squash Salad

Servings 6
Preparation and Cook time 40 minutes
INGREDIENTS:
- Red beetroots - 2, peeled and cubed
- Dried thyme - 1 tsp.
- Butternut squash - 1, peeled and cubed
- Extra virgin olive oil - 2 tbsp.
- Red onions - 2, quartered
- Salt and pepper - to taste
- Balsamic vinegar - 2 tbsp.

Directions:
1. Preheat oven to 350 degrees.
2. Put beetroots, squash, red onion, oil, salt, pepper and thyme in a deep baking dish and cook for 30 minutes.
3. Once cooked, pour all into a salad bowl and toss with vinegar. Eat salad warm from the oven.

Roasted pepper salad

Servings 4
Preparation Time 20 minutes
INGREDIENTS:
- Anchovy fillets - 4
- Lemon - 1, juiced
- Extra virgin olive oil - 1 tbsp.
- Garlic clove - 1
- Roasted red bell peppers - 8, sliced
- Pine nuts - 2 tbsp.
- Cherry tomatoes - 1 cup, halved
- Parsley - 2 tbsp., chopped
- Salt and pepper - to taste

Directions:
1. Ground lemon juice, olive oil, garlic and anchovies in a mortar and set aside for dressing.
2. Combine all other above **INGREDIENTS:** in a large salad bowl and then coat with the dressing mix.
3. Salad is ready to eat and should be served right away while fresh.

Pear salad with creamy yogurt dressing

Servings 4
Preparation Time 20 minutes
INGREDIENTS:
- Arugula - 4 cups
- Pears - 4, cored and sliced
- Walnuts - 1 2 cup, chopped
- Blue cheese - 2 oz., crumbled
- Plain yogurt - 1 4 cup
- Lemon juice - 1 tbsp.
- Extra virgin olive oil - 2 tbsp.
- Salt and pepper - to taste

Directions:

1. Using a jar or bottle, mix together lemon juice, yogurt, oil and salt and pepper to taste to make dressing, shaking well.
2. Now mix pears, blue cheese, sliced pears and walnuts in a separate, large salad bowl.
3. Lightly dress salad with yogurt mixture and eat immediately.

Watermelon Crunch Salad

Servings 4
Preparation Time 20 minutes
INGREDIENTS:
- Flat bread - 2, sliced
- Watermelon - 10 oz., cubed
- Feta cheese - 4 oz., cubed
- Cucumber - 1, sliced
- Extra virgin olive oil - 2 tbsp.
- Your choice of mixed seeds - 2 tbsp.

Directions:

1. Mix all of the above INGREDIENTS: in a bowl until well combined.
2. Once mixed, eat up!

Saved by the Bell Pepper Salad

Servings 4
Preparation Time 25 minutes
INGREDIENTS:
- Red bell peppers – 6, roasted and sliced
- Eggplant - 1, sliced
- Tahini paste - 2 tbsp.
- Chili flakes - 1 pinch
- Salt and pepper - to taste

Directions:

1. Mix all of your INGREDIENTS: together and add salt and pepper to suit your taste.
2. Serve and eat.

Summertime Salad

Servings 4
Preparation Time 25 minutes
INGREDIENTS:
- Tomatoes - 2, sliced
- Eggplant - 1, sliced
- Zucchini - 1, sliced
- Garlic cloves - 2, minced
- Red Onion - 2, sliced
- Balsamic vinegar - 2 tbsp.
- Dried mint - 1 tsp.
- Salt and pepper - to taste

Directions:

1. Take all of the vegetables (eggplant, onions, tomatoes and zucchini) and season with the salt and pepper to suit your taste.
2. Grill the veggies until they are brown.
3. Put grilled vegetables in a bowl with the garlic, vinegar and mint and mix together.
4. Serve up the salad as soon as mixed.

Best Beet Salad

Servings 4
Preparation Time 15 minutes
INGREDIENTS:
- Feta cheese - 3 oz., cubed
- Red beets - 6, cooked, peeled and sliced
- Balsamic vinegar - 2 tbsp.
- Extra virgin olive oil - 2 tbsp.

Directions:
1. Place sliced beets and feta cubes on a plate or platter.
2. Drizzle vinegar and oil over the top of beets and cheese and enjoy.

Parsley Spice Salad

Servings 2
Preparation Time 15 minutes
INGREDIENTS:
- Parsley - 2 cups, chopped
- Cumin powder - 1 4 tsp.
- Coriander seeds - 1 4 tsp.
- Chili powder - 1 4 tsp.
- Red wine vinegar - 1 tbsp.
- Cilantro - 1 4 cup, chopped
- Salt and pepper - to taste

Directions:
1. Mix all INGREDIENTS: in a salad bowl, except salt and pepper.
2. Use salt and pepper to season to suit your taste and then serve fresh.

Warm Broccoli Salad

Servings 4
Preparation and Cooking Time 20 minutes
INGREDIENTS:
- Extra virgin olive oil - 2 tbsp.
- Garlic cloves - 2, chopped
- Broccoli - 2 lbs., cut into florets
- Red pepper - 1, chopped
- Salt and pepper - to taste
- Capers - 1 tsp., chopped
- Green olives - 1 4 cup, sliced
- Cherry tomatoes - 1 cup, halved

Directions:
- Preheat oven to 350 degrees.
- Mix together garlic, broccoli, and oil in a baking dish and cook in oven for 10 minutes.
- Pour broccoli mix into a salad bowl and add in the remaining **INGREDIENTS:**.
- Mix well and add in salt and pepper to suit your taste. Salad should be serve while fresh.

Pancetta Cabbage Salad

Servings 4
Preparation and Cooking Time 20 minutes
INGREDIENTS:
- Cabbage - 1 head, shredded

- Parsley - 1 2 cup, chopped
- Red pepper - 1, chopped
- Green bell pepper - 1, cored and sliced
- Yellow bell pepper – 1, cored and sliced
- Red onion - 1, sliced
- Salt and pepper - to taste
- Apple cider vinegar – 2 tbsp.
- Pancetta - 2 oz., diced and fried

Directions:
1. Fry pancetta until crispy and set aside to cool.
2. Combine the cabbage, parsley, red pepper, bell peppers, red onion, salt and pepper in a salad bowl.
3. Mix all other INGREDIENTS: together in salad bowl and add in pancetta once it is cool.
4. This salad should be served fresh.

Insalata Caprese recipe

Preparation time: 15 minutes
Servings: 6
INGREDIENTS:
- extra virgin olive oil – 3 tbsps
- large ripe tomatoes – 4 (sliced 1 4 inch thick)
- black pepper to taste (freshly grounded)
- fresh basil leaves – 1 3 cup
- fine sea salt to taste
- pound fresh mozzarella cheese - 1 (sliced 1 4 inch thick)

Directions:
1. In an overlap and alternate manner, arrange on a large platter mozzarella cheese slices, tomato slices and basil leaves.
2. Add seasoning sea salt and pepper after drizzling with olive oil.

Orzo and Chicken Salad

Preparation time: 1h1 minutes
Servings: 4
INGREDIENTS:
- diced grilled chicken breast half – 1
- uncooked orzo pasta – ½ pound
- sprigs fresh oregano - 4
- olive oil – ¼ cup
- black olives – ¼ cup (cut in half lengthwise)
- red wine vinegar – 1 3 cup
- ground black pepper – ¼ tspn
- Dijon mustard – 1 tspn
- onion powder – ¾ tspn
- garlic powder – ¾ tspn
- dried basil – ¾ tspn
- salt – ½ tspn
- grape tomatoes – ½ cup (cut in half)
- crumbled feta cheese – 2 ounces
- red bell peppers – 2 (cut in half lengthwise and seeded)
- dried oregano – ¾ tspn

Directions:

1. In a big pot, fill with softly salted water and convey to a moving bubble over high warmth.
2. When the water is bubbling, mix in the orzo, and come back to a bubble.
3. Cook the pasta revealed, mixing at times, until the pasta has cooked through, yet is still firm to the chomp, around 11 minutes.
4. Channel well in a colander set in the sink, exchange to a bowl, and let cool in the fridge.
5. In a little bowl, whisk together the olive oil, red wine vinegar, Dijon mustard, garlic powder, oregano, basil, onion powder, salt, and pepper.
6. In a huge bowl, blend together the cooked orzo, tomatoes, olives, feta cheddar, and chicken bosom meat until altogether consolidated.
7. Pour the dressing over the orzo blend, softly blend to coat all fixings with dressing, and spoon into the red pepper parts.
8. Enhancement each presenting with an oregano sprig.

Delicious Tabbouleh

Preparation time: 2h10 minutes
Servings: 8
INGREDIENTS:

- peeled, seeded and chopped cucumber – 1
- chopped fresh mint – ¼ cup
- Bulgur – 1 cup
- boiling water – 1 2 3 cups
- olive oil – 1 3 cup
- chopped green onions – 1 cup
- salt – 1 tspn
- chopped fresh parsley – 1 cup
- ground black pepper to taste
- chopped tomatoes – 3
- lemon juice – 1 3 cup

Directions:

1. In a big bowl, combine boiling water with bulgur.
2. Set it aside after covering it to soak for 60 minutes.
3. Season to taste with black pepper and salt after addition of tomatoes, onions, oil, parsley, cucumber, mint and lemon juice; cover, refrigerate after tossing to combine for at least 60 minutes.

Mediterranean Chickpea

Salad **Servings:** 4
Preparation time: 20 minutes
INGREDIENTS:

- 15 ounce cooked chickpeas
- 1 Roma tomato seeded and diced
- 1/2 medium green bell pepper diced
- 1 tablespoon chopped fresh parsley
- 1 small white onion peeled and chopped
- ½ teaspoon minced garlic
- 1 lemon juiced
- 2 tablespoons olive oil

Directions:

1. Place all the INGREDIENTS in a bowl and toss until well mixed.

2. Cover the salad let chill for 15 minutes in the refrigerator and then serve.

Chickpea and Avocado Salad

Preparation time: 10 minutes
Cooking time: 30 minutes
Servings: 4
INGREDIENTS:
- 15 ounces canned chickpeas, drained
- Salt and black pepper to taste
- tablespoon extra-virgin olive oil
- avocado, pitted, peeled and chopped
- ½ teaspoon lime juice
- ounces feta cheese, crumbled
- scallions, chopped

Directions:
1. Place chickpeas on a lined baking sheet, add salt, pepper and oil, toss to coat, place in the oven at 400 degrees F and bake for 30 minutes.
2. In a bowl mix avocado with lime juice and mash well. Divide this between plates, add roasted chickpeas on top, salt, pepper, cheese and scallions and serve.

Nutrition Values: calories 230, fat 12, fiber 12, carbs 34, protein 13

Simple Mixed Herb Salad

Preparation time: 30 minutes
Cooking time: 0 minutes
Servings: 4
INGREDIENTS:
- tablespoons olive oil
- 1/3 cup tahini
- ½ cup raisins
- 4 tablespoons lemon juice
- 1 tablespoon water
- ¼ cup chives, chopped
- ¾ cup parsley, chopped
- ¼ cup cilantro, chopped
- Salt and black pepper to taste
- ¼ cup fennel, chopped
- ¼ cup dill, chopped
- ¼ cup mint leaves, torn radishes, cut into matchsticks
- ¼ cup pistachios, toasted
- ¼ cup tarragon, chopped 1 tablespoon sesame seeds, toasted

Directions:
1. Put raisins in a bowl, add warm water to cover, leave aside for 30 minutes, drain and put in a bowl.
2. In a small bowl, mix tahini with 3 tablespoons lemon juice, 3 tablespoons oil, salt, pepper and 1 tablespoon water and whisk well.
3. Arrange this on serving plates and leave them aside for now.
4. In a salad bowl, mix parsley with cilantro, chives, fennel, mint, dill, tarragon, remaining oil, the rest of the lemon juice, salt and pepper and toss to coat.
5. Divide this on tahini mix, top with raisins, pistachios, radishes and sesame seeds and serve.

Nutrition Values: calories 240, fat 22, fiber 2, carbs 18, protein 4

Grilled Potato Salad

Cooking time: 50 minutes
Servings: 6
INGREDIENTS:

- 4 sweet potatoes
- 3 tablespoons olive oil
- ¼ cup olive oil
- 1/3 cup orange juice
- 1 tablespoon orange juice
- 2 tablespoons pomegranate molasses
- ½ teaspoon sumac, ground
- 1 tablespoon red wine vinegar
- ½ teaspoon sugar
- Salt and black pepper to taste
- 1 tablespoon orange zest, grated
- 3 tablespoons honey
- 2 tablespoons mint, chopped
- 1/3 cup pistachios, chopped
- 1 cup Greek yogurt
- 1/3 cup pomegranate seeds

Directions:

1. Put potatoes on a lined baking sheet, place in the oven at 350 degrees F, bake for 40 minutes, leave them aside for 1 hour to cool down, peel them, cut into wedges and put on a cutting board.
2. In a bowl, mix ¼ cup oil with 1 tablespoon orange juice, sugar, vinegar, pomegranate molasses, sumac, salt and pepper and whisk.
3. In another bowl, mix the rest of the orange juice with orange zest, honey, salt, pepper and the remaining oil and whisk well again.
4. In a third bowl mix yogurt with some salt and pepper and with the mint and whisk. Brush potato wedges with the honey mix, add some salt, place on your kitchen grill pan heated over medium high heat, cook for 3 minutes and transfer to serving plates.
5. Sprinkle pistachios, pomegranate seeds, drizzle the vinaigrette, and serve with the yogurt sauce on top.

Nutrition Values: calories 240, fat 14, fiber 3, carbs 32, protein 5

Delicious Bread Salad

Preparation time: 10 minutes
Cooking time: 7 minutes
Servings: 4
INGREDIENTS:

- 1 shallot, chopped
- ¼ cup lemon juice
- 5 ounces bread, cubed
- ½ teaspoon sugar
- tablespoons olive oil
- Salt and black pepper to the taste
- 15 ounces canned chickpeas, drained
- 1/3 cup mint, chopped
- ounces cherry

- tomatoes cut in halves
- ounces feta cheese, crumbled
- 6 ounces snap peas, cut in quarters
- 3 ounces baby arugula

Directions:
1. Arrange the bread cubes in the oven at 350 degrees F, bake for 7 minutes and set aside to cool down.
2. In a bowl, mix sugar with shallot, lemon juice, salt and pepper, stir and set aside for 10 minutes.
3. Add the oil and mint and whisk well.
4. In a salad bowl, mix tomatoes with snap peas, chickpeas and the vinaigrette and toss to coat.
5. Add arugula, feta cheese, bread cubes, toss again to coat and serve right away.

Nutrition Values: calories 340, fat 23, fiber 12, carbs 23, protein 25

Potato Salad with Artichoke and Olives

Preparation time: 10 minutes
Cooking time: 20 minutes
Servings: 8
INGREDIENTS:
- ¼ cup lemon juice
- Salt and black pepper to the taste
- 2 teaspoons Dijon mustard
- ¼ cup olive oil
- 2 garlic cloves, minced and mashed
- ½ teaspoon red pepper flakes
- 2 teaspoons marjoram, chopped

For the salad:
- ¼ cup rice vinegar
- 1 tablespoon olive oil
- 3 and ¼ pounds baby red potatoes
- 2 cup frozen artichoke hearts
- Salt and black pepper to taste
- ¾ cup mint, chopped
- 1 cup black olives, pitted and chopped

Directions:
1. In a bowl, mix lemon juice with salt, pepper, mustard, ¼ cup oil, 2 garlic cloves, marjoram and pepper flakes and whisk well. In a bowl, mix vinegar with salt and whisk.
2. Put potatoes in a large saucepan, add salt and water to cover, bring to a boil over high heat, reduce temperature, cook for 10 minutes, take off heat, drain, cool them down, peel and cut them into chunks.
3. Put potatoes in a salad bowl, add rice vinegar mixed with salt and toss to coat.
4. Heat a pan with 1 tablespoon oil over medium high heat, add artichoke hearts and some salt and brown on both sides.
5. Add these over potatoes, then add mint and olives. Add salt and pepper to taste and the vinaigrette, toss to coat and serve.

Nutrition Values: calories 145, fat 4, fiber 3, carbs 11, protein 4

Veggie cheese salad

Served: 4
Preparation time: 25 minutes
INGREDIENTS:
- Chopped Parsley: 1 cup
- Chopped cilantro: 1 4 cup
- Pine nuts: 2 tablespoon
- 1 juiced lemon
- Chopped chives: 2 tablespoon
- 2 diced tomatoes
- C rumbled feta cheese: 4 oz.
- Chopped mint: 1 tablespoon
- Hot vegetable stock: 1 cup
- Couscous: 1 2 cup
- 2 Cooked and diced red beets
- Pine nuts: 2 tablespoon
- Pepper and salt as desired

Directions:
1. Combine the hot stock and couscous in a bowl and allow it to absorb all the liquid.
2. Pour in the cilantro, chives, tomatoes, beets, mint, Parsley and pine nuts.
3. Sprinkle pepper and salt as you wish, then pour in the lemon juice.
4. You can now top the salad with feta cheese and serve fresh.

Soft potato salad recipe

Servings: 6
Preparation time: 35 minutes
INGREDIENTS:
- Dijon mustard: 1 tablespoon
- 1 juiced lemon
- Extra virgin olive oil: 2 tablespoon
- New potatoes: 2 pounds
- Chopped dill: 2 tablespoon
- Red wine vinegar: 1 teaspoon
- Chopped parsley: 1 4 cup
- Chili flakes: 1 pinch
- Pepper and salt - to taste

Directions:
1. In a large pot, place the potatoes and cover with water.
2. Sprinkle in salt as desired and cook until the potatoes becomes soft.
3. After , drain them and cut into small chunks then transfer into a salad bowl
4. Pour in the dill, chili flakes and parsley In a bowl, mix the mustard, vinegar, lemon juice and oil.
5. Sprinkle pepper and salt as desired and mix well. You just prepared the salad dressing.
6. Pour the salad dressing over the potatoes then mix well. You can now serve the salad fresh.

Tomato rosemary salad

Servings: 4
Preparation time: 20 minutes
INGREDIENTS:

- Rice wine vinegar: 2 tablespoon
- 1 Finely chopped spring fresh rosemary
- Black pepper ground to paste
- 3 quartered large heirloom tomatoes
- Extra virgin olive oil: 1 4 cup
- 3 quartered small heirloom tomatoes
- Dried oregano: 1 8 teaspoon
- Kosher salt- to taste

Directions:

1. Mix the rice wine vinegar, oregano, olive oil and rosemary in a big bowl.
2. Add in the large and small tomatoes and shake until well coated.
3. Cover and refrigerate for 10-15 minutes until chilled.
4. Then season with black pepper and salt. Shake again.
5. You can now serve your salad fresh

Curry Salad

Preparation time: 20 minutes
Servings: 2
INGREDIENTS:

- Raisins – ¼ cup
- Grated sweet apple – 1
- chopped fresh parsley – 2 tbsps
- Grated carrots – 2

Dressing:

- maple syrup – ½ tsp or to taste (optional)
- Juiced lemon – 1
- curry powder – 1 tsp or more to taste
- olive oil – 2 tbsps
- ground black pepper and salt - to taste
- toasted sesame seeds – 1 tbsp (optional)

Directions:

1. In a bowl, add raisins, apple, parsley and carrots, raisins, and parsley together.
2. In a tight-fitting lid container or jar, mix maple syrup, sesame seeds, lemon juice, pepper, olive oil, curry powder and salt.
3. After covering the jar, shake till the dressing turn to a uniform yellow color.
4. Mix the dressing until it is evenly coated after pouring over salad.

Amazingly Fresh Carrot Salad

Serves: 4
Cook Time: 0 minutes
INGREDIENTS:

- ¼ tsp chipotle powder
- 1 bunch scallions, sliced
- 1 cup cherry tomatoes, halved
- 1 large avocado, diced

- 1 tbsp chili powder
- 1 tbsp lemon juice
- 2 tbsp olive oil
- 3 tbsp lime juice
- 4 cups carrots, spiralized
- salt to taste

Directions for Cooking:
1. In a salad bowl, mix and arrange avocado, cherry tomatoes, scallions and spiralized carrots. Set aside.
2. In a small bowl, whisk salt, chipotle powder, chili powder, olive oil, lemon juice and lime juice thoroughly.
3. Pour dressing over noodle salad. Toss to coat well.
4. Serve and enjoy at room temperature.

Nutrition Information: Calories per Serving: 243.6; Fat: 14.8g; Protein: 3g; Carbs: 24.6g

Asian Peanut Sauce Over Noodle Salad

Serves: 4
Cooking time: 10 minutes
INGREDIENTS:
- 1 cup shredded green cabbage
- 1 cup shredded red cabbage
- 1/4 cup chopped cilantro
- 1/4 cup chopped peanuts
- 1/4 cup chopped scallions
- 4 cups shiritake noodles (drained and rinsed)

Asian Peanut Sauce **INGREDIENTS:**
- ¼ cup sugar free peanut butter
- ¼ teaspoon cayenne pepper
- ½ cup filtered water
- ½ teaspoon kosher salt
- 1 tablespoon fish sauce (or coconut aminos for vegan)
- 1 tablespoon granulated erythritol sweetener
- 1 tablespoon lime juice
- 1 tablespoon toasted sesame oil
- 1 tablespoon wheat-free soy sauce
- 1 teaspoon minced garlic
- 2 tablespoons minced ginger

Directions for Cooking:
1. In a large salad bowl, combine all noodle salad **INGREDIENTS** and toss well to mix.
2. In a blender, mix all sauce **INGREDIENTS** and pulse until smooth and creamy.
3. Pour sauce over the salad and toss well to coat.
4. Evenly divide into four equal servings and enjoy.

Nutrition Information: Calories per serving: 104; Protein: 7.0g; Carbs: 12.0g; Fat: 16.0g

Blue Cheese and Arugula Salad

Serves: 4
Cooking time: 15 minutes
INGREDIENTS:
- ¼ cup crumbled blue cheese

- 1 tsp Dijon mustard
- 1-pint fresh figs, quartered
- 2 bags arugula
- 3 tbsp Balsamic Vinegar
- 3 tbsp olive oil
- Pepper and salt to taste

Directions for Cooking:
1. Whisk thoroughly together pepper, salt, olive oil, Dijon mustard, and balsamic vinegar to make the dressing.
2. Set aside in the ref for at least 30 minutes to marinate and allow the spices to combine.
3. 2) On four serving plates, evenly arrange arugula and top with blue cheese and figs.
4. 3) Drizzle each plate of salad with 1 ½ tbsp of prepared dressing.
5. Serve and enjoy.

Nutrition Information: Calories per serving: 202; Protein: 2.5g; Carbs: 25.5g; Fat: 10g

Chopped Chicken on Greek Salad

Serves: 4
Cooking time: 10 minutes
INGREDIENTS:
- ¼ tsp pepper
- ¼ tsp salt
- ½ cup crumbled feta cheese
- ½ cup finely chopped red onion
- ½ cup sliced ripe black olives
- 1 medium cucumber, peeled, seeded and chopped
- 1 tbsp chopped fresh dill
- 1 tsp garlic powder
- 1/3 cup red wine vinegar
- 2 ½ cups chopped cooked chicken
- 2 medium tomatoes, chopped
- 2 tbsp extra virgin olive oil
- 6 cups chopped romaine lettuce

Directions for Cooking:
1. In a large bowl, whisk well pepper, salt, garlic powder, dill, oil and vinegar.
2. Add feta, olives, onion, cucumber, tomatoes, chicken, and lettuce.
3. Toss well to combine.
4. Serve and enjoy.

Nutrition Information: Calories per serving: 461.9; Protein: 19.4g; Carbs: 10.8g; Fat: 37.9g

Classic Greek Salad

Serves: 4
Cooking time: 10 minutes
INGREDIENTS:
- ¼ cup extra virgin olive oil, plus more for drizzling
- ¼ cup red wine vinegar
- 1 4-oz block Greek feta cheese packed in brine
- 1 cup Kalamata olives, halved and pitted
- 1 lemon, juiced and zested
- 1 small red onion, halved and thinly sliced
- 1 tsp dried oregano

- 1 tsp honey
- 14 small vine-ripened tomatoes, quartered
- 5 Persian cucumbers
- Fresh oregano leaves for topping, optional
- Pepper to taste Salt to taste

Directions for Cooking:
1. In a bowl of ice water, soak red onions with 2 tbsp salt.
2. In a large bowl, whisk well ¼ tsp pepper, ½ tsp salt, dried oregano, honey, lemon zest, lemon juice, and vinegar. Slowly pour olive oil in a steady stream as you briskly whisk mixture. Continue whisking until emulsified.
3. Add olives and tomatoes, toss to coat with dressing.
4. Alternatingly peel cucumber leaving strips of skin on. Trim ends slice lengthwise and chop in ½-inch thick cubes. Add into bowl of tomatoes.
5. Drain onions and add into bowl of tomatoes. Toss well to coat and mix.
6. Drain feta and slice into four equal rectangles.
7. Divide Greek salad into serving plates, top each with oregano and feta.
8. To serve, season with pepper and drizzle with oil and enjoy.

Nutrition Information: Calories per serving: 365.5; Protein: 9.6g; Carbs: 26.2g; Fat: 24.7g

Coleslaw Asian Style

Serves: 10
Cook Time: 0 minutes
INGREDIENTS:
- ½ cup chopped fresh cilantro
- 1 ½ tbsp minced garlic
- 2 carrots, julienned
- 2 cups shredded napa cabbage
- 2 cups thinly sliced red cabbage
- 2 red bell peppers, thinly sliced
- 2 tbsp minced fresh ginger root
- 3 tbsp brown sugar
- 3 tbsp soy sauce
- 5 cups thinly sliced green cabbage
- 5 tbsp creamy peanut butter
- 6 green onions, chopped
- 6 tbsp rice wine vinegar
- 6 tbsp vegetable oil

Directions for Cooking:
1. Mix thoroughly the following in a medium bowl: garlic, ginger, brown sugar, soy sauce, peanut butter, oil and rice vinegar.
2. In a separate bowl, blend well cilantro, green onions, carrots, bell pepper, Napa cabbage, red cabbage and green cabbage.
3. Pour in the peanut sauce above and toss to mix well.
4. Serve and enjoy.

Nutrition Information: Calories per Serving: 193.8; Protein: 4g; Fat: 12.6g; Carbs: 16.1g

Cucumber Salad Japanese Style

Serves: 5 servings
Cook Time: 0 minutes
INGREDIENTS:

- 1 ½ tsp minced fresh ginger root
- 1 tsp salt
- 1/3 cup rice vinegar
- 2 large cucumbers, ribbon cut
- 4 tsp white sugar

Directions for Cooking:

1. Mix well ginger, salt, sugar and vinegar in a small bowl.
2. Add ribbon cut cucumbers and mix well.
3. Let stand for at least one hour in the ref before serving.

Nutrition Information: Calories per Serving: 29; Fat: .2g; Protein: .7g; Carbs: 6.1g

Easy Quinoa & Pear Salad

Serves: 6
Cooking time: 0 minutes
INGREDIENTS:

- ¼ cup chopped parsley
- ¼ cup chopped scallions
- ¼ cup lime juice
- ¼ cup red onion, diced
- ½ cup diced carrots
- ½ cup diced celery
- ½ cup diced cucumber
- ½ cup diced red pepper
- ½ cup dried wild blueberries
- ½ cup olive oil
- ½ cup spicy pecans, chopped
- 1 tbsp chopped parsley
- 1 tsp honey
- 1 tsp sea salt
- 2 fresh pears, cut into chunks
- 3 cups cooked quinoa

Directions for Cooking:

1. In a small bowl mix well olive oil, salt, lime juice, honey, and parsley. Set aside.
2. In large salad bowl, add remaining **INGREDIENTS** and toss to mix well.
3. Pour dressing and toss well to coat.
4. Serve and enjoy.

Nutrition Information: Calories per serving: 382; Protein: 5.6g; Carbs: 31.4g; Fat: 26g

Fruity Asparagus-Quinoa Salad

Serves: 8
Cooking time: 25 minutes
Salad **INGREDIENTS:**

- ¼ cup chopped pecans, toasted
- ½ cup finely chopped white onion
- ½ jalapeno pepper, diced

- ½ lb. asparagus, sliced to 2-inch lengths, steamed and chilled
- ½ tsp kosher salt
- 1 cup fresh orange sections
- 1 cup uncooked quinoa
- 1 tsp olive oil
- 2 cups water
- 2 tbsp minced red onion
- 5 dates, pitted and chopped

Dressing **INGREDIENTS:**
- ¼ tsp ground black pepper
- ¼ tsp kosher salt
- 1 garlic clove, minced
- 1 tbsp olive oil
- 2 tbsp chopped fresh mint
- 2 tbsp fresh lemon juice
- Mint sprigs – optional

Directions for Cooking:
1. Wash and rub with your hands the quinoa in a bowl at least three times, discarding water each and every time.
2. On medium high fire, place a large nonstick fry pan and heat 1 tsp olive oil. For two minutes, sauté onions before adding quinoa and sautéing for another five minutes.
3. Add ½ tsp salt and 2 cups water and bring to a boil. Lower fire to a simmer, cover and cook for 15 minutes. Turn off fire and let stand until water is absorbed.
4. Add pepper, asparagus, dates, pecans and orange sections into a salad bowl. Add cooked quinoa, toss to mix well.
5. In a small bowl, whisk mint, garlic, black pepper, salt, olive oil and lemon juice to create the dressing.
6. Pour dressing over salad, serve and enjoy.

Nutrition Information: Calories per Serving: 173; Fat: 6.3g; Protein: 4.3g; **CARBOHYDRATES**: 24.7g

Garden Salad with Oranges and Olives

Serves: 4
Cooking time: 15 minutes
INGREDIENTS:
- ½ cup red wine vinegar
- 1 tbsp extra virgin olive oil
- 1 tbsp finely chopped celery
- 1 tbsp finely chopped red onion
- 16 large ripe black olives
- 2 garlic cloves
- 2 navel oranges, peeled and segmented
- 4 boneless, skinless chicken breasts, 4-oz each
- 4 garlic cloves, minced
- 8 cups leaf lettuce, washed and dried
- Cracked black pepper to taste

Directions for Cooking:
1. Prepare the dressing by mixing pepper, celery, onion, olive oil, garlic and vinegar in a small bowl. Whisk well to combine.
2. Lightly grease grate and preheat grill to high.
3. Rub chicken with the garlic cloves and discard garlic.

4. Grill chicken for 5 minutes per side or until cooked through.
5. Remove from grill and let it stand for 5 minutes before cutting into ½-inch strips.
6. In 4 serving plates, evenly arrange two cups lettuce, ¼ of the sliced oranges and 4 olives per plate.
7. Top each plate with ¼ serving of grilled chicken, evenly drizzle with dressing, serve and enjoy.

Nutrition Information: Calories per serving: 259.8; Protein: 48.9g; Carbs: 12.9g; Fat: 1.4g

Grilled Eggplant Salad

Serves: 4
Cooking time: 18 minutes
INGREDIENTS:
- 1 avocado, halved, pitted, peeled and cubed
- 1 Italian eggplant, cut into 1-inch thick slices
- 1 large red onion, cut into rounds
- 1 lemon, zested
- 1 tbsp coarsely chopped oregano leaves
- 1 tbsp red wine vinegar
- 1 tsp Dijon mustard Canola oil
- Freshly ground black pepper
- Honey
- Olive oil
- Parsley sprigs for garnish
- Salt

Directions for Cooking:
1. With canola oil, brush onions and eggplant and place on grill.
2. Grill on high until onions are slightly charred and eggplants are soft around 5 minutes for onions and 8 to 12 minutes for eggplant.
3. Remove from grill and let cool for 5 minutes.
4. Roughly chop eggplants and onions and place in salad bowl.
5. Add avocado and toss to mix.
6. Whisk oregano, mustard and red wine vinegar in a small bowl.
7. Whisk in olive oil and honey to taste. Season with pepper and salt to taste.
8. Pour dressing to eggplant mixture, toss to mix well.
9. Garnish with parsley sprigs and lemon zest before serving.

Nutrition Information: Calories per serving: 190; Protein: 2.9g; Carbs: 16.7g; Fat: 12.4g

Kale Salad Recipe

Serves: 4
Cooking time: 7 minutes
INGREDIENTS:
- ¼ cup Kalamata olives
- ½ of a lemon
- 1 ½ tbsp flaxseeds
- 1 garlic clove, minced
- 1 small cucumber, sliced thinly
- 1 tbsp extra virgin olive oil
- 2 tbsp green onion, chopped
- 2 tbsp red onion, minced
- 6 cups dinosaur kale, chopped

- a pinch of dried basil
- a pinch of salt

Directions for Cooking:
1. Bring a medium pot, half-filled with water to a boil.
2. Rinse kale and cut into small strips. Place in a steamer and put on top of boiling water and steam for 5 – 7 minutes.
3. Transfer steamed kale to a salad bowl.
4. Season kale with oil, salt, basil and lemon. Toss to coat well.
5. Add remaining **INGREDIENTS** into salad bowl, toss to mix.
6. Serve and enjoy.

Nutrition Information: Calories per serving: 92.7; Protein: 2.4g; Carbs: 6.6g; Fat: 6.3g

Tomato Salad

Servings: 4
Preparation time: 20 minutes
INGREDIENTS:
- One cucumber, sliced
- ½ Cup black olives
- 1 pound cubed tomatoes
- ¼ Cup sun-dried tomatoes, chopped
- One red onion, sliced
- One tbsp balsamic vinegar
- ¼ Cup parsley, chopped
- Salt and pepper to taste
- Two tbsp olive oil

Instructions:
1. In a bowl combine all vegetables.
2. Add seasoning, vinegar and olive oil then stir well.
3. Mix well and serve the salad fresh.

Nutrition Value: Calories: 126 Fat: 9.2g Protein: 2.1g **CARBOHYDRATES**: 11.5g

Spiced Parsley Salad

Servings: 2
Preparation time: 5 minutes
INGREDIENTS:
- 2 Cups parsley (chopped)
- ¼ Cup cilantro (chopped)
- ¼ tsp cumin powder
- ¼ tsp chili powder
- ¼ tsp coriander seeds
- One tbsp red wine vinegar
- Salt and pepper to taste

Instructions:
1. In a bowl, combine all **INGREDIENTS**.
2. Adjust seasoning to taste and serve. Enjoy.

Nutrition Value: Calories: 26 Fat: 0.6g Protein: 1.9g **CARBOHYDRATES**: 4.2g

Mediterranean Salad

Servings: 5
Preparation time: 5 minutes
INGREDIENTS:

- 1 pound sliced tomatoes
- One sliced cucumber
- ½ Cup parsley (chopped)
- One sliced fennel bulb
- Salt
- One sliced red onion
- ¼ Cup sliced almonds
- One tsp dried oregano
- Black pepper
- ¼ Cup cilantro (chopped)
- One tbsp balsamic vinegar
- One juiced lemon
- Two tbsp olive oil

Instructions:

1. In a bowl combine all vegetables.
2. Add seasoning, vinegar and olive oil then stir well.
3. Serve and enjoy.

Nutrition Value: Calories: 107 Fat: 7.0g Protein: 2.7g **CARBOHYDRATES**: 10.7g

Watermelon Feta Salad

Servings: 2
Preparation time: 15 minutes
INGREDIENTS:

- 16 oz. seedless watermelon, cubed
- 4 oz. feta cheese, crumbled
- Two tbsp extra virgin olive oil
- One tsp chopped thyme

Instructions:

1. In a bowl, combine the watermelon and feta.
2. Sprinkle oil and thyme before serving. Enjoy.

Nutrition Value: Calories: 339 Fat: 26.4g Protein: 9.4g **CARBOHYDRATES**: 19.7g

CPSIA information can be obtained
at www.ICGtesting.com
Printed in the USA
BVHW051051150221
600147BV00011B/784